Gutbliss

Gutbliss

A 10-DAY PLAN TO BAN BLOAT, FLUSH TOXINS, AND DUMP YOUR DIGESTIVE BAGGAGE

Robynne Chutkan, MD, FASGE

AVERY
a member of Penguin Group (USA)
New York

Published by the Penguin Group
Penguin Group (USA) LLC
375 Hudson Street
New York, New York 10014

USA · Canada · UK · Ireland · Australia
New Zealand · India · South Africa · China

penguin.com
A Penguin Random House Company

Recipes courtesy of Elise Museles of Kale and Chocolate (www.kaleandchocolate.com).
Reprinted with permission.

"Sweet Breathing" (page 237) courtesy of Emily Perlman, MS, BCB.
Adapted from Richard Gevirtz and Paul Lehrer.

Most Avery books are available at special quantity discounts for bulk purchase for sales
promotions, premiums, fund-raising, and educational needs. Special books or book excerpts also
can be created to fit specific needs. For details, write: Special.Markets@us.penguingroup.com.

Library of Congress Cataloging-in-Publication Data

Chutkan, Robynne.
Gutbliss : a 10-day plan to ban bloat, flush toxins, and dump your
digestive baggage / Robynne Chutkan, MD, FASGE.
p.   cm.
ISBN 978-1-58333-522-2 (hardback)
1. Gastrointestinal system—Diseases—Diet therapy.   2. Digestive organs—
Diseases—Popular works.   3. Women—Health and hygiene—Popular works.
4. Cooking for the sick.   I. Title.
RC816.C48   2013   2013024823
616.3'30654—dc23

Printed in the United States of America
1   3   5   7   9   10   8   6   4   2

BOOK DESIGN BY TANYA MAIBORODA

To my darling Sydney:

May you find everything you need for

abundantly good health in the garden and on the mat.

All disease begins in the gut.

—HIPPOCRATES

Contents

PART 1

Digestion 101

PART 2

What's Gone Wrong in Your Gut?

PART 3

On the Path to Gutbliss

Acknowledgments

GUTBLISS STARTED OUT AS A BOOK ABOUT FOOD. I WAS ALARMED BY what I was seeing in people's digestive tracts and the growing prevalence of bloating and other gastrointestinal complaints. To me, food was the obvious but frequently overlooked connection. So I set out to write a book about how our food was making us sick. Along the way, I had the incredible good fortune to meet Howard Yoon, my literary agent, who helped me mold my passion about food and the gut into a broader conversation that included the obstacles to digestive wellness and how to go about removing them. Whether you like this book or not (and I hope you do!), it is undoubtedly a much better one because of Howard's wisdom, patience, and belief that I had something important to say. And for the opportunity to say it, I am eternally grateful to Lucia Watson and Bill Shinker at Gotham/Avery, to Gabrielle Campo, who guided me through the entire process, and to Toni Sciarra Poynter, who provided invaluable editorial assistance.

To my husband, Eric, who at this point knows far more than he ever imagined he would about bowel movements and gut bacteria, and whose support never wavered as I abandoned my post for several months at a time to focus on completing this book. Without his encouragement and overall picking up of the slack at home this book would never have been possible. And to my amazing daughter, Sydney, who loves to talk about bowel movements and gut bacteria, and who spent so many hours keeping me company in my study while this manuscript was being written. You are a constant source of inspiration.

Bette Greenhause and I have been keeping company since my first day on the job at Georgetown in 1997. Without her, the Digestive Center for Women would never have come to fruition. I do not think I could practice medicine without her. To the late Dr. Henry Janowitz and Dr. Jerry Waye, who taught me much about both the art and the science of gastroenterology. To Gena Hamshaw, whose journey from editor to doctor I am honored to be a part of. To all my friends who put up with canceled dinners and no-shows while I wrote this book and cheered me on toward the finish line. A special thank-you to Dr. Ida Bergstrom, Alicia Sokol, Jill Hudson, and Elise Museles. Vernon Jordan, Doug Heater, and Robert Raben are my three wise men. I am grateful to them for always pointing me in the right direction. To my parents, for teaching me the invaluable lesson that with good living comes mostly good health.

A huge thank-you to Dr. Mehmet Oz, for giving me the opportunity to share my passion for digestive wellness with America. And most of all, to the many patients along the way, who have taught me so much. It has been an honor and a privilege.

Introduction

"WHY AM I SO BLOATED?" THAT'S A QUESTION I HEAR NEARLY EVERY DAY in my gastroenterology practice. Over the course of my medical career, I've gone from helping a handful of women a week with bloating, sluggish fullness, and constipation to feeling like I'm dealing with a full-on epidemic. For many, the symptoms are daily, relentless, and life altering, but even when they're not that severe, they're always annoying.

The causes of bloating vary tremendously, from common benign conditions to rare, life-threatening illnesses. Some may be connected to behaviors you don't even think about. (Do you talk with your mouth full? You could be swallowing enough air to go up a dress size!) Some you may have heard of but need more information and aren't quite sure whether you should be worried. (Is celiac disease the same as gluten intolerance?) Some may surprise you. (Taking antacids to settle your stomach can make your jeans un-zippable!) In this book you'll learn about these issues and many more, including how to tell if your bloating is serious . . . or if you're just seriously bloated.

Your Inner Doctor

The information in this book incorporates aspects of both conventional and alternative medicine to create an intuitive, commonsense approach to digestive wellness. The goal is not to scare you into having an unnecessary procedure or taking a pill you don't need, but to encourage you to explore the cause of your symptoms and to implement some useful basic strategies, many of which are already in your toolbox.

I believe that buried deep beneath the information overload we all receive from consumer marketing is our own innate sense of what we need to make ourselves well. I like to call it our "inner doctor." This book will help you access that deep inner sense, building your understanding by providing reliable information on what helps and what hinders when it comes to your digestive health.

Many digestive problems that a decade ago we thought were "all in people's heads" we now know are caused by very real gastrointestinal disturbances—conditions like bacterial overgrowth and gluten intolerance. I refuse to believe that millions of women who suffer from bloating but don't have a diagnosis are "crazy" or "just stressed out." I've seen how often, by thinking outside the box, we're able to find both the problem and the remedy.

I want to help you trust your inner doctor. If you think there's something going on, there probably is, and you need to keep searching till you find the right person who can help you figure it out. They may not always have a white coat on and an MD behind their name. Much of what I know I've learned from patients, nutritionists, biofeedback practitioners, holistic health coaches, naturopathic doctors, acupuncturists, farmers, and even my yoga instructor. I hope the information in this book will serve as a guide to help you understand what's going on in your body and offer you some real solutions.

My Promise to You

I've spent a lot of time inside the digestive tract, observing what's gone wrong and why. This book contains the information I think is most important to share, in short, digestible (pardon the pun) chapters. When I don't know something, I'll tell you I don't know. When I think a particular practice is shady or suspect, I'll tell you that, too. I'll give you the information that has been helping my patients make real improvements in their digestive health—including a comprehensive 10-Day Gutbliss Plan to heal yourself from the inside out, based on twenty years of experience. It's helped thousands of women tighten their tummies and end their discomfort. Many have reported a surge in energy and mood, too! This easy-to-follow integrative approach to digestive wellness will help you banish bloat, flush toxins, and dump your digestive baggage—the healthy way.

The world these days can be an intimidating place. We worry about environmental toxins, drugs can be dangerous, and Mother Nature would hardly recognize much of what's available at the grocery store. But left to its own devices, the human body is still a marvel, with an amazing capacity to recover and heal itself, particularly when injurious practices are identified and stopped. My sincere hope is that you're able to use the information in this book to find your own gutbliss and that when you and I meet, it'll be at the farmer's market or on the yoga mat, and not in my office.

Finding My Gutbliss

In 2004 I decided to leave the hallowed halls of academia and set up my own practice. Georgetown Hospital had been my first job when I finished my training in New York in 1997, but after almost eight years, hospital-based medicine no longer seemed to have the answers my patients and I were looking for. I owed a lot to the institution—my career had flourished there: I had a sixteen-page résumé of published articles, book chapters, and speaking engagements throughout the United States and Europe; I had helped to train over thirty gastroenterologists; I had colleagues I respected and admired; and I enjoyed the teaching opportunities. My salary was more than generous. My professional life was bountiful and I should have been happy, but I wasn't. I had lost my faith.

Over the years my priorities had gradually shifted from high-tech procedures that diagnose and treat disease to no-tech lifestyle modifications that prevent them. It was becoming difficult for me to emphasize the industry message in my speaking and teaching that colonoscopy saves lives (which it does) without giving equal billing to what I had come to believe:

that diet and lifestyle were more important in achieving and maintaining digestive health than any procedure I could recommend. Philosophically, I felt a lack of alignment. I was interested in an integrative and more holistic approach to digestive diseases and I wanted that to be part of my message. My colleagues seemed more interested in technical innovation. Their mission and approach hadn't changed, but mine had.

The practice of gastroenterology had also changed and was feeling more and more like a business venture, with the patients as the consumers and endoscopy as the product. Many gastroenterologists now owned their own endoscopy units, as well as the pathology services used to process their biopsy specimens. While this allowed for better quality control and closer collaboration, it also greatly incentivized doctors to do more procedures and biopsies.

The gastroenterologists I knew were people who cared deeply about their patients, but many of them struck me as overly committed to doing procedures. I wanted to provide patients with equally relevant lifesaving information—like the fact that switching to a plant-based diet can cut your risk for colon cancer in half; or that exercise and a low-fat diet can prevent gallstones—not just perform procedures.

A screening colonoscopy takes from fifteen to thirty minutes to perform. The reimbursement to the physician when done in an outpatient facility that they own can be several times what they make for an office visit of the same length. It's not hard to do the math and see why the nature of my specialty was changing. The economics simply don't encourage problem solving and exploration beyond the endoscope.

At the same time that gastroenterologists are being incentivized to do more procedures and spend less time talking to patients, the nature of digestive illnesses is changing, too. We're seeing more conditions related to diet, lifestyle, and environmental factors, and diagnosing and treating those conditions requires more than just a quick endoscopy.

Not all gastroenterologists are singularly focused on the revenue stream that endoscopic procedures like colonoscopies provide. Many have the kind of medical practices that embrace more integrative solutions, educating their patients about the importance of dietary intervention and other preventive measures, and exploring alternative diagnoses, while performing endoscopy in a responsible manner.

But providing comprehensive digestive care is not always easy or straightforward. It requires extra time for us to sit down and talk with patients about what they're eating and how they're living. It requires research into things we're unfamiliar with, and consideration of the possibility that maybe our colleagues in the alternative medicine world know a thing or two. That kind of care means a lot of additional education in things we learned nothing about in medical school and that we can't touch and see with our endoscopes.

Thanks to the Internet, some patients know more about their digestive disorder than their gastroenterologist, although they may not have the tools and context that allow them to manage it. So they're turning to their yoga instructors, massage therapists, life coaches, and social network for medical advice. Visits to alternative practitioners outnumber visits to conventional doctors four to one, even though they usually aren't covered by insurance. Conventional gastroenterology, while flourishing in the realm of advanced procedures and screening of healthy populations, is falling short in providing people with what they really need: reliable information on how to achieve and maintain digestive wellness.

I knew these were vitally important issues that needed to be addressed with patients. But I was still spending most of my time doing procedures and prescribing complicated drugs with lots of side effects. My philosophy had changed; now my practice needed to change, too.

An Integrative Solution

In 2004, while pregnant with my first child and renovating a house down to the studs, I decided to open a practice that was more in line with my philosophy of an integrative approach to digestive disease. In addition to providing patients with resources in nutrition, stress reduction, and exercise, there were three basic principles I wanted to adhere to:

1. Ensure sufficient time with my patients to explore problems in detail.
2. Abide by my belief that most people aren't crazy, even if their symptoms don't always make sense.
3. Make and keep a commitment to think outside the box.

I gave notice at Georgetown, found an ideal location, applied for a tax ID number, and opened my doors. I called the practice the Digestive Center for Women, although it turns out women aren't the only ones interested in more integrative solutions to their digestive troubles, and men constitute about 20 percent of our patients. I remained a voluntary faculty member at Georgetown and continued to perform procedures at the hospital, although the number of procedures was much lower than what I had previously been doing.

Slowly but surely, patients came.

Many of them had already been evaluated and diagnosed by very competent gastroenterologists. They didn't come because I was smarter than their last doctor; they came to have a dialogue and to get ideas and feedback on what they could do to improve their digestive health. We talked in detail about symptoms, test results, nutrition, and stress and the possible relationship among them. I didn't always have the answers, but I usually knew where to look.

I built an integrative practice that relied a great deal on the excellent skills of my collaborators: a biofeedback practitioner, integrative nutritionists, exercise physiologists, and referrals to practitioners in counseling, acupuncture, and massage.

I continued to see patients with complex problems related to Crohn's disease and ulcerative colitis, which had been my area of expertise at Georgetown. I found that these patients, too, benefited greatly from an integrative approach that included nutritional intervention and stress reduction.

My focus shifted from scientific papers in medical journals on the role of endoscopy to articles in yoga, health, and women's magazines on the role of diet and lifestyle in preventing and treating digestive diseases. My talks at national gastroenterology meetings were now about obesity and the gastroenterology practice of the future, which would incorporate cooking classes, biofeedback, meditation workshops, and exercise sessions, not just endoscopy facilities.

I was grateful for the opportunity to merge my personal beliefs with my professional practice and engage a larger audience with what I believed to be the truth about digestive health. I decided to write a book to share what I had learned over the years about how to achieve a blissful gut, and I enthusiastically began work on the outline and manuscript.

On the last day of my tenure on the governing board of the American Society for Gastrointestinal Endoscopy (ASGE), I pitched an idea for a nonprofit called Gutrunners, which would focus on improving digestive health through educating the public about the benefits of nutrition and exercise. I was delighted when the ASGE agreed to be the founding sponsor and provided a loan as seed money. Gutrunners incorporated as a nonprofit in the state of Maryland and I dove into my new role as executive director, race director, and fund-raiser, arranging races at national gastroenterology conferences and meeting with potential sponsors and participants. Life was very busy but filled with meaningful work that I loved.

Bliss*less*

I had witnessed firsthand with many of my patients what happened when work-life balance was disrupted, but, ironically, I failed to see the warning signs in my own life.

Although my practice was incredibly rewarding, the decrease in the number of lucrative procedures relative to what I'd been doing at Georgetown and the fact that I was in solo practice (i.e., there was no one with whom to share expenses) meant a drop in income.

My days at the office were long and I spent my nights working on the book, writing articles, and trying to get Gutrunners off the ground. It was thrilling to have founded an organization dedicated to the principles I believed in, but now I was responsible for running it, and in the hole personally for the loan amount, which was to be repaid to the ASGE within five years.

My schedule was a brutal six a.m.-to-midnight routine that was difficult to maintain. My leisurely daily runs and regular yoga practice fell by the wayside. I now only had time for occasional weekend warrior workouts that left me sore the next day and did little to improve my fitness level. My daughter was the joy of my life, but there was never enough time with her.

I had grown up eating fresh produce from my grandfather's farm and home-cooked meals every day and had continued those traditions in our household. But now dinner was frequently takeout and not always healthy. I didn't have time for lunch most days and was eating way too much sugary and starchy food for quick energy. Some days half my calories came from cookies. The more sugar I ate, the more of it I craved, and my consumption increased dramatically. I'm not a coffee drinker so sugar became my caffeine, causing wide swings in my mood and blood sugar, which left me feeling even more tired.

I also started drinking champagne at night while I worked. I'd not been much of a drinker in college, medical school, or the years since, but as life got busier and more stressful, it became part of my routine to have a glass or two after dinner. The sugar in the champagne was what attracted me. It opened the floodgates for more cravings, so there was often a sweet dessert happening along with the champagne. The late nights and excessive sugar gave me a terrible headache the next day and left me bleary-eyed and exhausted.

Here I was, preaching attention to proper nutrition, leisure, stress reduction, and exercise to my patients—and I was having a hard time practicing what I preached.

Out of Balance

I'd never had any serious medical problems, and my only experience as a patient had been with labor and delivery, so I was unprepared for poor health when it finally arrived. And because I still thought of myself as a healthy person with good habits, it took me a while to recognize what was going on.

For the first time in my life, I was bloated. And constipated. It gets worse: I had persistent rectal itching at night that drove me absolutely crazy. At first I thought the itching was from a hemorrhoid, but close inspection proved that diagnosis to be incorrect. Then I was sure it must be pinworms, since night itching is a characteristic symptom, but that wasn't what I had, either.

Other symptoms that I developed included rosacea (misdiagnosed as acne), chronic sinus infections, fatigue, brain fog, dark circles under my eyes, thinning hair, a ten-pound weight gain, food intolerances (especially to dairy and nuts), and body odor. I know this last one is somewhat subjective, but even after running ten miles or doing ninety minutes of hot yoga, my sweat had previously been profuse but odorless.

I looked and felt terrible. And despite all my knowledge, or maybe because of it (a subconscious belief that sickness happens to other people, not to us, can be a common trait among physicians), it took me several months to figure out the diagnosis. I had severe bacterial imbalance, also known as dysbiosis. My starchy, sugary diet, excessive dessert, after-dinner champagne, lack of exercise, and skyrocketing stress had altered the delicate balance of "good" and "bad" bacteria in my gut, and I was experiencing the fallout. My less-than-healthy diet and lifestyle had changed my entire body chemistry, and the results were manifest both internally (bloating and constipation) and externally (rosacea and hair thinning). After a sugar binge I could feel my face burning as the rosacea flared and the rectal itching became unbearable as the yeast in my body multiplied. Clumps of hair filled the shower drain, and I was exhausted all the time.

As varied and disparate as they seemed, my symptoms were all a result of dysbiosis, except for the brain fog and episodes of extreme fatigue, which turned out to be manifestations of gluten sensitivity.

How I Found My Gutbliss

As disconcerting as it was to lose control of my own health, the experience was valuable and meaningful. It affirmed some of the difficult choices I'd made about the kind of medical practice I believed in and highlighted a lot of the shortcomings of gastroenterology as it's practiced today. Dysbiosis can't be detected or treated with an endoscopic procedure. It's the sort of diagnosis that can only be made through a careful evaluation of someone's history, as well as the ability to recognize the relationship among a number of ostensibly unrelated symptoms. It's a condition that might easily escape conventional detection and be written off as stress or anxiety.

In this book, you'll learn a lot more about dysbiosis and how to recognize and address it. Having firsthand experience with a condition like this has given me a renewed sense of purpose. It has made me more confident than ever that the future of medicine depends on doctors' willingness to listen, to use food and fitness as tools in the pursuit of health, and to think outside the proverbial prescription and procedure box. Lifestyle-related conditions such as dysbiosis significantly disrupt your quality of life yet can't be detected through a standard procedure. They represent the new kind of digestive illness so prevalent today. Dysbiosis and conditions such as food allergies, leaky gut, parasitic infections, candida overgrowth, gluten intolerance, and many others can lead to frustration and self-doubt for undiagnosed patients stumbling around in the dark looking for answers.

Even after I realized the cause of my symptoms, it took me a while to implement the changes I needed to feel better. Despite my good dietary foundation of fruits and vegetables, the addictive nature of some of the not-so-healthy food I was eating had taken hold, and it was hard to let go. I continued to experiment with gluten, avoiding it for several days and then eating a bagel to see what would happen. Invariably the symptoms of brain fog and intense fatigue would return. I'd do well avoiding dessert and alcohol during the week but continued to indulge on the weekends, paying the price with an increase in symptoms and the slow burn of suboptimal health.

The strategy that ultimately worked for me was to finally completely eliminate the foods I knew were causing my symptoms and affecting my health. It was easy to identify what those foods were: I felt awful after consuming them, and they were the same culprits responsible for many of my patients' digestive problems. Incremental change may seem like less of a challenge, but it can be hard to maintain because it takes a while before you experience a tangible difference in your symptoms, and so people frequently give up. I knew from experience with my patients that it took about ten days for a dietary change to be experienced physically and also for it to become psychologically easier to maintain. Withdrawal symptoms from sugar and other carbohydrates are the most prominent in the first week and then tend to become less intense. Going through the process of habit change myself helped me better understand and help my patients as they did the same.

I found my gutbliss by getting rid of GAS: gluten, alcohol, and sugary treats. I also slowed things down a little at work and at home and rediscovered the healthful habits that had previously sustained me. Green juices instead of champagne kept me company at night, and a few pieces of dark chocolate became my new splurge. I had more energy in the mornings to start running and practicing yoga again, and my daughter took on the role of sous-chef as we spent time together in the kitchen whipping up healthy meals. With the help of a good probiotic, more kale than I ever thought I could eat, regular exercise, and eliminating GAS, the dysbiosis and all its symptoms gradually improved and I got back to looking and feeling healthy and strong. These days I enjoy the occasional dessert, croissant, or glass of champagne, but I pay attention to how I nourish myself, and my diet, as well as my digestive tract, feels balanced and joyful.

The Journey Continues . . . Together

Gutbliss is truly a journey, not a destination, and I continue to explore what feels best and is the right path for me. There's still lots on my to-do list, including deepening my yoga practice, completing a full Ironman Triathlon, experimenting with veganism, moving my gastroenterology practice to a farm, and learning to play the guitar, but I appreciate where I am and the good health that I have right now.

We live differently but we suffer similarly. My sincere hope is that if you're suffering from bloating or any form of digestive distress, you'll find your gutbliss within the pages of this book.

PART 1

Digestion 101

1

What's Happening in There?

YOUR GASTROINTESTINAL (GI) TRACT IS THE ENGINE FOR YOUR ENTIRE body. Your cells depend on the nutrients extracted there from the food you eat for energy and on other essential ingredients like oxygen and minerals they need to survive. It's an incredibly complex and specialized system, and every part plays a crucial role.

There are multiple points along this thirty-foot digestive superhighway where things can go awry. Bloating is one of the earliest and most common indications that there may be a problem. In this chapter I'll give you a quick overview of the digestive system and some of the things that can go wrong along the route. The more familiar you are with your GI tract, the easier it is to determine whether you've taken a wrong turn somewhere along the way.

A Trip Down Your Digestive Superhighway

GI discomfort can start at any point in the digestive tract, from the mouth to the anus and everywhere in between. The upper GI tract includes the mouth, esophagus, stomach, and the first part of the small intestine called the duodenum. Digestion actually begins in the mouth, where enzymes in saliva start to break down food. Gravity and muscular contractions help propel things down the long tubular esophagus into the stomach, where hydrochloric acid provides the optimum pH for digestive enzymes such as pepsin to break down protein and other food molecules.

Alcohol, caffeine, nicotine, fatty foods, and a too-full stomach can all send acid back up into the esophagus where it doesn't belong and leave you reaching for antacids—which, it turns out, may not be such a great idea. Stomach acid is a crucial part of the digestive process. Decreasing acid production with medications can lead to major problems, including poor absorption of nutrients and overgrowth of harmful bacteria, which is a major cause of bloating. Delayed emptying of the stomach, called gastroparesis, can bloat you, too. It's an underdiagnosed condition associated with nausea and abdominal pain that can lead to vomiting and weight loss in severe cases.

Once semi-digested food known as chyme has passed through the stomach, digestion continues in the small intestine. This is where our bodies start to extract the nutrients from food. Coming out of the stomach, chyme is very acidic, but the small intestine secretes a hormone called cholecystokinin (CCK), which stimulates the gallbladder to release alkali bile into the intestines, changing the acid content. Bile helps with the digestion of fats by providing a detergent-like effect, which emulsifies the fats so that they can dissolve in liquid and be more easily absorbed through the lining of the GI tract. Too much fat in the diet can cause gallstones, a problem that's frequently blamed on the gallbladder and leads to surgery. Although we can live without our gallbladder, digestion is never the same without it.

As the food breaks down into smaller and smaller molecules, it's absorbed across the surface area of the small intestine by tiny fingerlike projections called villi. Conditions like celiac disease flatten your villi and can lead to bloating, malabsorption, and lots of other problems. The absorbed nutrients are transported via the bloodstream to the liver, the main detoxification organ in the body. In addition to removing toxins from the blood, the liver synthesizes hormones, proteins, and bile.

Your pancreas is a gland that also makes and secretes important hormones like insulin and pancreatic juice that contains enzymes crucial to the digestive process. Insulin helps glucose get from the bloodstream into

Bloating: Getting the Story Behind the Symptom

Symptoms like bloating are very nonspecific, and that can pose a real problem in pinning down a diagnosis. Any number of conditions can cause it, from garden-variety constipation to cancer. Look up "bloating" on the Internet and you're as likely to come up with a worrisome but unlikely diagnosis like pancreatic cancer as you are to find a probable explanation like lactose intolerance, leaving you confused and scared as to what might really be going on. With bloating, the symptom itself may not be as helpful as the story behind the symptom. That's why you have to make sure that the information you give your doctor is complete, with all the details, and that it's heard, that key questions are asked, and, most of all, that the person you're telling your story to believes that you know when something is not quite right with your body, even if you don't know exactly what it is. That's ultimately what will help you turn your bloating into a meaningful diagnosis that you can do something about.

the cells of your body to be used for energy. Insufficient amounts of insulin lead to diabetes, a serious illness characterized by high levels of glucose in the blood and not enough in the cells. The main digestive enzymes are proteases, amylases, and lipases; they digest protein, carbohydrates, and fat, respectively. Enzyme levels decrease with age, and chemicals in the food we eat and medications can decrease them even further, leading to maldigestion and bloating.

Wavelike contractions called peristalsis transport the products of digestion through the small intestine into the colon. One of the main functions of the colon is to absorb water from the stool into the bloodstream as it transports things to the finish line. When it's working well, water is extracted as the products of digestion move through the colon in a clockwise direction from right to left, and as a result the stool that comes out of the anus is solid. The colon is also the site of bacterial fermentation of unabsorbed materials. Lots of factors can affect the transit time and consistency of the stool and result in bloating and a change in bowel habits.

The things you can't see in the digestive tract may be more important than those you can. The trillions of bacteria and other organisms that live there play a crucial role in digestive health, as do the levels of digestive enzymes and hormones. That's why knowing which foods and habits upset the ratio of helpful to undesirable species and how to boost enzyme activity and optimize hormonal secretion is essential information.

Mechanical blockages, out-of-control hormones, bacterial imbalance, low enzyme levels, active inflammation, structural abnormalities, and a host of other issues can disrupt the smooth functioning of your digestive engine and lead to bloating and abdominal distress. It's vitally important to pay attention to the feedback your GI system gives you—what makes it feel good and what aggravates it. You'll be learning about this in later chapters. Over time, as you're able to read your digestive road map, you'll be able to figure out the changes and adjustments you need to keep your GI tract functioning like the miraculously efficient system it's meant to be.

2

The Voluptuous Venus Colon

ANNE IS A WISP OF A WOMAN WHO'S BEEN TERRIBLY BLOATED AND CON-
stipated for as long as she can remember. Two tablespoons of psyllium
husk (soluble plant fiber that adds bulk to the stool) and one tablespoon of
ground flax seed in the morning, followed by two capfuls of a polyethylene glycol osmotic cathartic (a powerful laxative), plus three stool soften-
ers and six prunes at night—and she still has difficulty having a bowel
movement. She's had several visits to the emergency room after nearly
passing out from abdominal pain. Each time, the main finding on X-ray
was a colon full to the brim with stool. We take a dietary history. Impec-
cable: she's quasi-vegetarian and her standard lunch is brown rice, lentils,
and kale. She's two years shy of being the age for a colon cancer screening,
and given the findings on X-ray, I recommend a colonoscopy to make sure
there's no obstructing lesion inside her colon.

On the day of the procedure, the anesthesiologist gets Anne nice and
comfortable, and within a few minutes she's asleep and I begin my journey
through her colon. I find this procedure fascinating, even after performing thousands of them, because just as every patient is unique, so every
colon is unique in its own way.

Anne's colon is an impressive maze of twists and turns and switchbacks and loops that are very difficult to navigate. After more than three times the amount of time it usually takes me to complete a colonoscopy, we are finally finished. The diagnosis: a voluptuous Venus colon.

Physiology, Not Psychology

Women may be from Venus and men from Mars, but are our colons really that different? It turns out that they are. As science in recent years has proven repeatedly, women aren't just smaller versions of men, and that means in the GI tract, too. There are significant anatomical differences in the female digestive tract that explain why bloating is such a problem for us.

In the medical literature there are lots of articles about colonoscopy being more difficult in women, requiring more sedation, and the procedure overall taking longer. The differences have been attributed to a lower pain threshold in women—something I find hard to believe, given the fact that most women go through labor without any anesthesia and the world's population is still growing. Anatomical variances between the female colon and her male counterpart are the real explanation for these differences, and for the significantly higher prevalence of constipation and bloating in women compared to men.

The Link Between Women and Bloating

Women tend to have longer colons than men, on average four to five inches longer. The difference is probably to allow for more absorption of fluids during pregnancy. Most of the extra female colon, which is sometimes referred to as a redundant, tortuous, or spastic colon, is in the transverse segment or low down in the sigmoid colon. Not only does the extra length predispose to loop formation during colonoscopy, making the procedure more challenging, but it's also prone to loop formation at other times, too, particularly when the colon is filled with gas or stool. When the products of digestion get stuck in these sharp angulations, there's a lot of gas buildup behind the blockage, leading to tremendous discomfort and bloating.

It was episodes like this that had landed Anne in the emergency room.

The pain from the stretching of a full segment of colon led to what's called a vasovagal reaction in which her heart rate dropped and she felt sweaty, nauseated, and dizzy. It's a reaction I've seen in lots of people with extreme constipation and bloating when the colon gets too full of stool or gas, or after colonoscopy if too much air is left in the colon.

In addition to a longer colon, women have a more rounded, deeper pelvis than men. The combination of the shape of the pelvis and the added length of the colon causes the colon to drop deep into a woman's pelvis, where it competes for space with her ovaries, Fallopian tubes, uterus, and bladder. This can lead to a lot of looping, crowding, constipation, and bloating. By contrast, men's reproductive organs take up much less space, and their narrower pelvis doesn't usually lead to the bowel taking up residence there. A visual representation of the male colon would be a gentle horseshoe shape, while the female visual would be a Six Flags roller coaster.

Hormonal differences play a role, too. Higher levels of testosterone in men result in an abdominal wall that's generally more muscular and defined, which buttresses the colon, preventing it from forming redundant loops and keeping things moving through more efficiently. Even men with a beer belly often have a relatively tight abdominal wall underneath, which is why they'll complain about being fat but not bloated. In addition to less testosterone, women sometimes have too much estrogen on board, a condition called estrogen dominance that's associated with the growth of uterine fibroids and endometriosis, both of which can press on the bowel and be a major source of bloating. (Surgical removal of the uterus, a common treatment for fibroids and endometriosis, is also a risk factor for bloating because of the scar tissue that can develop afterward in the abdominal cavity, hampering the colon's freedom of movement and creating additional angulations and kinks.)

Anne was thrilled to hear she didn't have colon cancer or any other worrisome condition inside her colon. As it turned out, some of the positive things she was doing needed some tweaks to help maximize their benefits. She was eating large amounts of fiber, but she was doing it at one sitting. This was contributing to her bloating as the bulky stools were getting stuck in the hairpin turns of her colon, causing a lot of discomfort. She modified her diet to keep her total intake of fiber the same, but she spread it out throughout the day. She also doubled up her water consumption to help move the fiber through her digestive tract more efficiently. As a result, she was able to stop taking the stool softener and osmotic cathartic at night.

Just knowing the diagnosis was tremendously helpful to Anne in managing her symptoms. When she felt her bowels getting backed up and started to become really bloated, she'd do a liquid diet for a day, drinking primarily green veggie juices and broth, sometimes with a couple of doses of the cathartic to help clean things out. Her colon still required a lot of attention, but there were no more near-fainting spells or trips to the emergency room.

On occasion I've had to prescribe a full bowel prep for patients with a voluptuous Venus colon filled with stool, but I always recommend not letting things get to that point by doing a day or two of liquids, instead of blasting your bowels with osmotic cathartics.

A longer colon, a deeper pelvis, a less defined abdominal wall, and hormonal influences—all of these factors can conspire to constipate and bloat us. But knowing what's going on inside can help you manage your bloat—including figuring out when to lighten up your diet to give your curvy colon a chance to decompress.

3

Traffic Jams on the GI Superhighway?

AS MENTIONED IN CHAPTER 1, THE GASTROINTESTINAL TRACT IS ONE long road, from the mouth to the anus. There are no shortcuts, bypasses, or alternate routes—and unfortunately, there can be plenty of obstacles along the way, both structural and functional. In this chapter we'll look at some of the conditions that slow things down en route and can be a major source of bloating. I'll also provide you with some useful information on what to do if your digestive contents are stuck in transit.

Expect Delays

Deborah had been complaining of severe bloating, abdominal pain, and heartburn for a few months, which was worse after meals. She had tried over-the-counter antacids and prescription acid suppressors to no avail. She didn't have any of the common risk factors associated with acid reflux that cause heartburn: she was a nonsmoker, didn't drink caffeine, and wasn't overweight. Her job with a large international bank meant lots of time sitting in meetings, but she went running every evening after work and did yoga on the weekends. Dinner at around nine p.m. was her main meal, since breakfast was light and lunch nonexistent. Her husband did most of the cooking, and dinner was meat, chicken, or fish with a starch and a vegetable, and sometimes a glass of wine and a piece of chocolate for dessert.

Deborah was worried about an ulcer and so was I, since she took a lot of nonsteroidal anti-inflammatory drugs (NSAIDs) for aches and pains from running. These medications are notorious for causing ulcers and inflammation in the GI tract, so I scheduled her for an endoscopy to take a look.

When I sedated Deborah and inserted the endoscope through her esophagus into her stomach, I was very surprised by what I saw: no ulcers and a normal stomach, but a large mound of what looked like cheese and tomato sauce sitting right in the middle of everything.

The first thing I asked Deborah when she woke up was whether she had forgotten to fast before the procedure and had eaten breakfast by mistake. No, she had dutifully followed the written instructions. Her last meal had been cheese pizza the night before at nine p.m. The fact that I could still see it sitting in her stomach eleven hours later was definitely not normal.

To confirm my suspicions, I sent Deborah for a test called a gastric emptying study that measures how long your stomach takes to empty after eating. You're given food containing a small amount of radioactive material, and your stomach is scanned from the outside to see how long it takes for the food to pass through. Less than half of it should be in the stomach at the completion of the test.

Deborah's results were very abnormal: at the end of the test, 80 percent of the food was still in her stomach!

The gastric emptying study confirmed Deborah's diagnosis: delayed emptying of the stomach, a condition called gastroparesis, which means partial paralysis of the stomach. The stomach isn't really paralyzed in gastroparesis, but its function is slowed down to varying degrees and bloating is one of the most common symptoms.

We don't know the reason behind gastroparesis in most people. The vagus nerve, which controls stomach emptying, can be damaged or affected by illness, causing the muscles to not work properly. Diabetes, intestinal surgery, narcotic medications, some antidepressants, and neurological conditions like Parkinson's disease and multiple sclerosis are causes. It can also occur after certain viral illnesses.

Fatty Foods, Too Full of Fiber, and Sleepy Stomachs: Lifestyle Causes of Gastroparesis

Gastroparesis can be severe in some people, especially in diabetics, whose stomach emptying can completely shut down when their blood sugar is poorly controlled, leading to pain, bloating, and recurrent episodes of vomiting after eating. In most people, the symptoms are much less severe and usually fluctuate, with flare-ups that can be precipitated by a large fatty meal or by eating too much fiber in one sitting.

Deborah had originally thought her symptoms were due to reflux, and, in fact, lots of people with reflux have an element of gastroparesis that contributes to their symptoms. Reflux happens when the valve between the esophagus and stomach that should be shut tight when food isn't passing into the stomach opens inappropriately, allowing partially digested food and acid to enter the esophagus. Caffeine, alcohol, and nicotine can all cause the valve to open, but a full stomach that's not emptying properly can also force the valve open, causing reflux symptoms in addition to the discomfort of a fully stretched stomach.

People with gastroparesis usually complain of bloating, abdominal pain, and feeling abnormally full after eating, particularly with meals containing a lot of fat. Fat takes longer to digest than other kinds of food, so when receptors in the stomach sense a high fat content, they send a signal to the nerves that control emptying to slow down even more. That's why even small amounts of fatty foods like duck breast or bacon are really filling, even for those of us without gastroparesis.

Because high-fiber foods can be filling, they, too, can be problematic in gastroparesis. That's why I recommend splitting them up into small servings. Avoiding carbonated beverages is also helpful.

In addition, Deborah needed to rethink her meal schedule. She felt like she'd swallowed a bag of bricks after meals, especially dinner, which was by far her largest meal. Because she ate so little during the day, she'd still be hungry after dinner and would continue to snack until she went to bed at midnight. By then she was extremely bloated and could feel the food just sitting there for hours. Occasionally after a large, rich meal, she'd be so uncomfortable she'd make herself vomit.

You may not know that your stomach actually has a bedtime. Its muscular contractions are tied to the light-dark cycle, also known as the circadian rhythm. Contractility is most active during the day, when the sun is up, and least active at night, after it sets—which is unfortunately when most of us consume the majority of our calories. To make matters worse, after filling our sleepy stomach with food at night, we usually recline on the sofa or bed, so we don't have the benefit of gravity and movement to help transport things from north to south. Eating large meals at night is sure to bloat you and make gastroparesis worse, and it can also cause or exacerbate reflux.

I told Deborah that although there were some medications that could help improve the contractility of her stomach, most of them were poorly tolerated, with side effects that included neurological symptoms. The good news was that there was a lot we could do with her diet, starting with some calorie shifting and imposing a strict curfew on nighttime eating. The new guidelines were: breakfast like a queen, lunch like a princess, dinner like a pauper—and nothing to eat after nine p.m.

The main problem was her running schedule and what to do about dinner. She got terrible cramping and nausea if she ran within a few hours after eating. She had no idea why this happened, but she had stopped eating lunch in order to accommodate her evening run. Now we knew her cramping and nausea were the result of her delayed emptying: she was essentially running with a stomach full of food even though it was hours after eating.

Deborah wasn't a morning person, but she agreed to try running before work a couple of days a week. On those days, the plan was to eat a big breakfast after her run, a good-sized lunch, and a light dinner at seven p.m. instead of nine p.m., since she had already gotten her run out of the way. On the days she planned to run in the evening, she split her calories up into mini-meals. The first one was a medium-sized breakfast before she left the house, followed by a snack at around ten a.m. Then came a light lunch at noon, and a piece of fruit at one p.m. This still gave her six hours between her last mouthful and her seven p.m. run. She ate dinner right after running, usually soup or a salad that her husband had prepared, not waiting to eat until after her shower, as she had previously been doing.

One of the biggest changes for Deborah was her morning routine. I don't believe that you have to eat breakfast first thing in the morning if you don't have an appetite, as long as you have something nutritious available when you do start to get hungry. Deborah wasn't hungry in the mornings because she was still full from all the food she had eaten late the night before. Once we reset things with a much lighter dinner at an earlier time and no eating after nine p.m., she found she actually had an appetite for breakfast, particularly on her morning run days. She also found she could tolerate relatively fatty foods much better early in the day than at night, so breakfast was sometimes leftover dinner, which included the occasional slice of pizza.

If you have symptoms of gastroparesis and feel poorly after eating, one of the things that will make it worse is skipping meals, because it almost always leads to overeating later in the day. Your body needs a minimum number of calories to perform its activities of daily living. If you don't provide them during the day when it needs them, it will send you in search of them at night, when you don't. Eating small, frequent meals (making sure you don't go too long in between eating) is an important part of getting your symptoms under control. Travel with food and make sure you always have a healthy, low-fat snack like a piece of fruit with you. When offered the choice, go out for lunch rather than dinner. You'll tolerate a restaurant meal better during the day and feel less hungry at night. Don't fill your stomach up with too much liquid during meals either; hydrate in between meals instead. Although liquids generally empty much faster than solids, they can still fill you up and bloat you. Even chugging water after exercise can precipitate symptoms, so if you're prone to delayed emptying, take your time hydrating post-workout with frequent small sips.

The other important piece of advice is to move around as much as you can, especially after eating. You don't need to run a marathon after meals; even a quick walk around the block will help to stimulate peristalsis and get your stomach moving, especially after nighttime or large meals. Going for an evening constitutional after dinner is a great tradition to establish.

If you have gastroparesis, you probably already figured out that the worst thing you can do is to eat a large, fatty meal late at night and then hop right into bed. If you don't have gastroparesis, eating a large, fatty meal late at night and then hopping right into bed will also slow down your stomach emptying and make you feel sick, so it's sage advice either way.

Medical Issues That Can Slow Things Down

Gastroparesis can slow things down significantly, but some conditions can bring digestion to a standstill, causing severe bloating.

ADHESIONS

If you've had previous abdominal or pelvic surgery, even if it was many years ago, you may have developed scar tissue in your abdomen or pelvis. Scar tissue can cause cobweb-like adhesions that trap loops of bowel and can cause a complete or partial bowel obstruction. A complete obstruction causes severe pain as the segment of bowel above the blockage stretches and tries to push things through. If the obstruction isn't relieved, the bowel can burst open, causing a perforation, which is a medical emergency.

A partial obstruction will cause bloating and pain, but things will still be able to pass through, and the symptoms might be more chronic. If you think adhesions may be the cause of your bloating, you should definitely have a medical evaluation. An X-ray or CAT (computerized axial tomography) scan of the abdomen may not show the scar tissue, but it may reveal air-filled, dilated loops of bowel above the level of the blockage. For people who are having recurrent episodes of obstruction, surgical exploration of the abdomen to look for and remove scar tissue is usually the next step.

VOLVULUS

Volvulus is a mechanical condition that can cause severe intermittent bloating. It occurs when the bowel twists abnormally onto itself, causing obstructive symptoms that can become severe if the twisting compromises the blood supply. It usually occurs low down in the colon in the sigmoid section, especially in older sedentary people or in those with a long, redundant colon.

RADIATION

A history of radiation to the abdomen or pelvis can also cause obstructive symptoms like bloating and pain, either through the formation of scar tissue or by radiation damage to the bowel itself. The symptoms may occur within a few months of the radiation or may appear years or even decades after.

PSEUDO-OBSTRUCTION

Chronic intestinal pseudo-obstruction, sometimes called Ogilvie's syndrome, causes symptoms that mimic a bowel obstruction, but without any mechanical cause. It usually occurs in people with lots of other serious illnesses, or after surgery, and can cause massive dilation of the colon.

HERNIA

The abdominal wall is like a bandage that straps the bowel down and keeps it from bulging out. A defect in the wall from a hernia, which is like a tear in the bandage, and can be associated with previous abdominal surgery, pregnancy, and weight lifting, can cause bloating that's constant or intermittent. Loops of bowel can become trapped in the hernia and cut off from their blood supply, which is a medical emergency that leads to dead bowel if not remedied surgically. Hernias can occur anywhere in the abdomen or groin. Coughing or bearing down to have a bowel movement will often result in the bowel bulging out through the hernia. If you're having pain in addition to bloating and think you have a hernia, you should definitely get it checked out to avoid the possibility of incarcerated or trapped bowel.

DIASTASIS RECTI

Diastasis recti is a gaping space in the midline of the rectus abdominus muscle, the large, prominent muscle located in the center of your abdomen that separates it into right and left halves. The condition occurs primarily in pregnant or postpartum women as a result of stretching of the muscle by the enlarged uterus, and can also occur in newborns when the muscle isn't fully developed at birth. Although most textbooks say it's primarily a cosmetic condition, like hernias, diastasis recti can be a major cause of bloating because of the defect in the abdominal muscle, which would normally bind the bowel in place.

TUMORS OR OTHER MASSES

A tumor or mass from another organ that presses on the bowel is one of the more worrisome causes of bloating and obstructive symptoms. Sometimes the lesion is benign, as in the case of endometriosis, uterine fibroids, or ovarian cysts, but sometimes it's something more serious, like pancreatic or ovarian cancer. We'll discuss some of these more ominous causes of bloating in Chapter 18, "Seriously Bloated."

Or Maybe Your Superhighway Is a Country Road?

Some people just have slow transit, and you may be one of them. If you're experiencing delays, there are lots of things you can do to help get your digestive products to their final destination in a timely fashion.

Gutbliss Solutions to Keep Traffic Moving

If you think you could have gastroparesis, a hernia, volvulus, scar tissue, diastasis recti, tumor, bowel obstruction, or some other serious condition that's causing symptoms, it's important to get a thorough evaluation and a clear diagnosis. For those with milder symptoms or a country road kind of superhighway, here are some tips that can help alleviate symptoms and keep things moving:

- **Don't skip meals.** It invariably results in overeating later in the day when the stomach is even less active.
- **Eat small, frequent meals.** Your stomach is about the size of your fist. It can be stretched to a much larger capacity, but this often results in pain and nausea. Eating mini-meals every three to four hours will keep you from getting hungry while also giving your stomach adequate time to empty in between meals.

- **Split servings.** Consider taking your usual meal and splitting it into two servings a few hours apart.
- **Pack snacks.** Travel with snacks like a piece of fruit to avoid going for long periods of time without eating.
- **Calorie shift.** Eat your largest meal early in the day when your stomach is most active and your smallest meal at night: breakfast like a queen, lunch like a princess, and dinner like a pauper.
- **Eat out early.** If you're going to eat out, make it lunch or brunch rather than dinner.
- **Impose a dinner curfew.** Stomach contractility decreases markedly after dark, so stop eating at sunset, or shortly thereafter.
- **Wait four hours after eating to exercise or lie down.** This will ensure you're not jogging or sleeping with a full stomach.
- **Go for a walk after meals.** Movement encourages peristalsis and will help hasten stomach emptying.
- **Watch out for fatty foods.** Limit your consumption of foods with a high fat content, such as meat, cheese, and cream sauces, which slow down stomach emptying.
- **Split up your fiber consumption.** Avoid eating a large amount of fiber at one time, which can lead to a full stomach and abdominal discomfort.
- **Sip, don't gulp.** Hydration is important for keeping the products of digestion moving, but don't chug large amounts of fluid. Sip on fluids throughout the day instead. Drink liquids in between rather than during meals to avoid overfilling the stomach.

Getting Regular

CONSTIPATION IS ONE OF THE MOST COMMON COMPLAINTS IN MY PRAC-
tice, and it's one I love to treat because there's almost always a satisfying solution. Since constipation and bloating are often fellow travelers, treating one often leads to resolution of the other. In this chapter I'll talk about what can cause constipation and how it might be contributing to your bloat. I'll also share my favorite remedies for getting things moving.

Ancient Problem, Common in Modern Life

The ancient Egyptians believed in the concept of autointoxication: stagnating stool in the colon that could result in toxins being absorbed through the lining into the bloodstream, ultimately poisoning the body. They also believed that hardened feces that accumulated along the lining of the colon could lead to the overgrowth of what we now refer to as harmful bacteria and interfere with the absorption of water and nutrients. If you've ever suffered from serious constipation, you know that a colon full of stool can make you feel like you're poisoned: bloated, sluggish, and toxic. These days, constipation is more common in Western societies due to a diet that's low in fiber and high in processed food, dairy, and meat.

Diagnosis and Causes: A Tricky Business

There are lots of different criteria for diagnosing constipation. Most are based on stool consistency, whether evacuation is complete, and the number of stools—fewer than three per week being the standard textbook definition. But the fact is that you can have a bowel movement every day and still be constipated. I see patients who move their bowels regularly but always feel full and uncomfortable. On exam I can feel bowel loops filled with stool that feel like fat sausages. So while there's an official guideline for diagnosis, a lot has to do with how the patient feels. Sometimes people who are squeezing out a stingy stool every day may not even realize they're constipated until they come to me for problems with bloating—and are pleasantly surprised when a constipation fix also solves their bloating woes.

Constipation is a symptom, not a disease, and there's always at least one explanation, and sometimes three or four, for why it's happening. That's why I'm prone to peppering people with questions about size, shape, consistency, ease of passage, and even the odor of their bowel movements. They're all important clues about why things aren't moving: small pebbly stool might mean diverticulosis; toothpaste-thin stool could be a sign of colon cancer but also occurs commonly with diverticulosis; layered concretions that look like they've been deposited at different times could suggest a problem with contractility of the colon; painful passage with bleeding could be a fissure; a foul smell could mean a parasite or bacterial overgrowth, both conditions that typically cause loose stools but can also have the opposite effect. Figuring out the underlying reasons for your constipation and coming up with the right remedy may take a bit of detective work, but when your bowels start to function like a well-oiled machine, it's a wonderful thing.

What's Happening Down There?

Chances are you haven't thought much about this, but if you're serious about your health, it really is important to know how bowel movements (and constipation and bloating) happen as part of understanding and caring for this amazing body of yours.

The products of digestion move through the bowels, becoming more solid as they pass through the colon, from right to left, and are ultimately deposited in the sigmoid colon and rectum. In textbooks the sigmoid is depicted as a gentle S, but in reality it looks more like a badly tangled Slinky, especially in women, where it competes with the pelvic organs for space. The voluptuous curves of the sigmoid can hold a lot of stool—days' and even weeks' worth. In some constipated people, new stool is deposited at the top of the sigmoid every day while the stool at the bottom is excreted. The remaining column of stool in between that gets left behind is the sausage roll I can feel when I palpate their abdomen.

Bloating: Constipation's Frequent Companion

Nothing's worse for ruining your gutbliss than being constipated, and if you're constipated, chances are you're also bloated. These two go hand in hand for a couple of reasons. If you're constipated, you likely have one of the following (or both): you're either plugged down below, or you have slow transit where things just aren't moving through fast enough.

Obstructed defecation, the technical term for being plugged, may have mechanical or functional causes, the commonest being a large, hard wad of stool. Slow transit can be caused by diet, inactivity, medications, hormonal changes, or systemic problems like diabetes and hypothyroidism.

In Chapter 1, "What's Happening in There?" we talked about the GI tract being a thirty-foot-long superhighway. It starts at the mouth and ends at the anus. If there's a roadblock along the way, there's no detour to take—it's one road from start to finish. That can mean a major pileup and serious bloating, not only from things not moving through, but from bacteria in the colon fermenting the stagnating stool for longer than normal, causing increased gas production . . . and bloating.

How Bowel Movements Happen

Most of the constipation I see involves a backup of stool in the rectum, the very end of the colon. In order to understand what can go wrong down there, it's helpful to understand a bit about the rectum's anatomy and physiology.

The rectum is essentially a reservoir that stores stool before it exits through the anus. It's about six inches long, with a diameter of one-and-a-half to two inches.

Normally the rectum is very distensible, like a balloon. You may feel the urge to go in the morning but decide to wait until the afternoon (something I absolutely recommend against). The rectum can easily expand to hold the stool without any problem. How good is the rectum at holding stool? Really good: the threshold volume at which most people can feel stool in their rectum is about 20 milliliters, but the maximum tolerated volume is 400 milliliters, which is a lot of stool.

Two sphincters that wrap around the rectum like a sheath are primarily responsible for the important tasks of keeping stool in and getting it out. The internal anal sphincter (IAS) is the innermost sheath and is under involuntary control, like your blood pressure or heart rate. It's difficult to consciously influence it, although biofeedback and relaxation techniques can help when the need arises. Normally the IAS is in a contracted state, keeping things closed tight to prevent leakage, and relaxing when stool has to come out. The external anal sphincter (EAS) is the outermost sheath and is under voluntary control. Like moving your hands or feet, you can relax or contract it at will, depending on whether you're trying to have or prevent a bowel movement.

Defecation is the process of having a bowel movement, and it involves both voluntary and involuntary actions. As stool fills the rectum, it expands until it reaches the threshold volume that triggers stretch receptors in the wall to initiate contraction. The IAS relaxes while the EAS contracts. The sphincters send a signal to the brain that it's time to defecate, and the brain sends a signal back to the rectum coordinating movement of the necessary muscles. The abdominal muscles contract, increasing pressure in the abdomen, which helps to force the stool out, and the perineum (the genitals and anus) drops down toward the toilet. The puborectalis muscle loops around the rectum like a sling and is normally in a contracted state, creating a bent ninety-degree angle between the rectum and the anal canal that helps to hold stool in. During defecation the puborectalis relaxes and the angle between the anal canal and the rectum straightens out, providing a straight shot for stool to pass out. As the rectum contracts to empty its contents, peristaltic waves help force the stool out.

As you can see, something that we do thousands of times in our lifetime actually takes a lot of coordination between different parts of the body, including the central nervous system, autonomic nervous system, and chest, respiratory, abdominal, and pelvic muscles. Moving waste products out of the body is *that* important. Even the amount of blood pumped by the heart decreases when you're having a bowel movement. Diet; activity level; hormones; medications; and anatomical, neurological, and psychological factors all play a role in keeping things moving.

What Can Go Wrong

There are multiple areas where things can run amok, as evidenced by the 2.5 million doctor visits per year and up to 60 million people in the United States who are constipated. Here are some of the commonest and most problematic causes.

HOLDING

One of the most important things you can to do to prevent constipation is to heed your body's call to move your bowels when it first happens. Ignoring that signal and holding stool in when it's trying to come out causes all sorts of problems, including something called reverse peristalsis, where stool is pushed back up into the colon. The low pressure in the rectum now that the stool has migrated back up means that the stretch receptors won't trigger contraction, decreasing your chances of having a bowel movement anytime soon. The longer you hold the stool in, the more water is extracted from it and the harder it gets. You also totally confuse the sphincters and puborectalis muscles that are now being clenched tight, despite signals from the central nervous system that they should be relaxed and opening.

One of the first questions I ask constipated patients is whether they were holders when they were younger, meaning, when they felt an urge to go, did they frequently ignore it? This is common in girls, who tend to be more fastidious about where they use the bathroom. Kids spend a lot of their time at school where the bathroom situation is usually far from ideal: the facilities sometimes aren't that clean, they're not that private (you can see through the space between or under the doors), you can hear and smell what's going on, there may or may not be toilet paper, there's constant anxiety about boys coming in, and concern about finishing in time to get to class. Not to mention the utter panic if you have an urgent call during class and you have to raise your hand and ask—out loud—for permission to go to the bathroom. Basically, everybody knows your intimate business at a time when far more innocuous things embarrass most kids. Many of my patients tell me they never, ever used the bathroom at school, allowing reverse peristalsis to flourish as unheeded urges forced stool in the wrong direction.

SHY BOWEL

When I was a gastroenterology fellow in New York, I had a friend who was very particular about where she used the bathroom. She was dating an actor who had a Fifth Avenue penthouse with eight bathrooms, but she would take a cab back to her apartment to have a bowel movement. They spent a week together in the Caribbean, and she refused to have a bowel movement the entire time, lest he hear, see, or smell it. The vacation ended with a trip to the emergency room for fecal impaction, the technical term for being full of stool. She suffered from parcopresis, otherwise known as shy bowel: an inability to have a bowel movement without a certain level of privacy.

Shy bowel is different from the normal embarrassment many people have about bowel movements, and the need for safe places to move their bowels can impose severe lifestyle limitations. The privacy requirement can vary. Some people can't have anyone else in the same house or apartment or even the same building.

One of my patients with very challenging constipation endured a trauma in childhood that permanently affected her ability to have normal bowel movements—she was in the middle of doing her business in the woods on a camping trip when she was discovered by the rest of the campers, including several boys. Decades later, she still has a hard time unclenching her sphincter. The feeling of shame associated with moving her bowels was firmly established, and from then on she had terrible parcopresis. She could only have bowel movements in absolute privacy, with no one around, including her husband and children. She would wait until the middle of the night when everyone was asleep to furtively use the bathroom, not even flushing until morning for fear of being discovered. Defecating at work, in a restaurant, or when her family was awake was totally out of the question. It took lots of biofeedback and therapy to retrain her muscles to allow her to feel relaxed enough in the bathroom to allow the stool to exit when her safe haven conditions were not entirely met.

ANISMUS

Anismus is a frequent but underdiagnosed cause of constipation and bloating. It goes by a lot of different aliases: dyssenergic defecation, inappropriate puborectalis contraction, puborectalis syndrome, paradoxical puborectalis, pelvic floor disorder, spastic pelvic floor syndrome, and anal sphincter dyssenergia. All refer to the same thing: the pelvic floor muscles don't relax when you're trying to have a bowel movement. This makes getting the stool out very challenging. In addition to constipation and bloating, people with anismus may also complain of tenesmus (a feeling of incomplete evacuation), and a need to insert a finger into the rectum or vagina or push on the perineum in order to extract stool.

Dehydration and inactivity are risk factors for anismus, but holding and anxiety about bowel movements are also common causes. An anal fissure that causes pain with the passage of stool can also be a cause. A lot of people diagnosed with garden-variety constipation actually have anismus. Laxatives and bulking agents typically don't bring relief unless the lack of muscle relaxation is addressed, too. In fact, people with undiagnosed anismus may get worse when prescribed high doses of fiber because now they're plugged with a bigger plug and their pelvic muscles still aren't relaxing—making them feel even more bloated and uncomfortable. They're often frustrated and hopeless about their inability to have a normal bowel movement, and their social life may suffer because they feel chained to the toilet.

So how do we diagnose anismus? Anorectal manometry can help. It involves inserting a balloon catheter into the rectum and having the patient squeeze and push. The catheter is connected to a machine that records the pressure associated with these various maneuvers and determines whether appropriate relaxation is taking place.

Defecography is another useful test. It provides X-ray images of contrast material given by enema as it travels through the rectum and anal canal. It tells us if the rectum is emptying properly and can identify structural issues that may be causing a problem.

Although these are useful tests, most people aren't in a hurry to have a balloon in their rectum or be X-rayed while they try to push contrast material out. The good news is that if you have anismus, your gastroenterologist may be able to figure it out just from your history and what they find on rectal exam, if they can get you to relax enough. When they ask you to bear down like you're having a bowel movement, if you have anismus your gastroenterologist should be able to feel your muscles tightening around their finger instead of relaxing. Sometimes just inserting a finger is difficult because the muscles are so tight. Although most people don't look forward to that part of the visit, a good rectal exam can provide important clues about the cause of your constipation.

RECTAL PROLAPSE, INTUSSUSCEPTION, AND RECTOCELE

A good rectal exam can also pick up mechanical problems associated with straining and bloating. Here are the ones you should know about:

- Rectal prolapse: the rectum protrudes out through the anus, usually as a result of chronic straining and constipation. Usually occurs with bowel movements but can also be present in the absence of defecation.

- Rectal intussusception: sometimes known as internal rectal prolapse. This happens when the top part of the rectum telescopes down into the lower part or into the anal canal, causing a blockage. More common in women due to damage to the pelvic floor during childbirth.
- Rectocele: the wall of the rectum bulges into the vagina, which is directly in front of it, as a result of a weakness in the wall—usually from long-standing constipation or pressure during a vaginal delivery. Stool can get stuck in a rectocele, and women will often figure out that inserting a finger into their vagina and pressing backward on the wall of the rectum helps to get the stool out. Although this can be embarrassing information to volunteer, it's important to let your doctor know, because if you do this on a regular basis the diagnosis is likely a rectocele or a pelvic floor problem (see "Pelvic Floor Disorders" below), and there are things that can be done to improve it. One important point: if you have a rectocele associated with anismus, the lack of relaxation of the pelvic muscles needs to be addressed before any kind of corrective surgery for the rectocele is contemplated so the problem won't recur.

PELVIC FLOOR DISORDERS

Pelvic floor disorders are what happen when things literally start to go south. The rectum, bladder, uterus, and vagina are supported by muscles and connective tissue that keep them in place, sort of like a hammock that everything rests on. Pregnancy, straining, large-birth-weight babies, gynecological surgery, and aging can all weigh the hammock down, creating weakness in the pelvic floor. Urine leakage is the most common complaint, but stool leakage or constipation can also develop. Kegel exercises to strengthen the muscles are helpful, as is biofeedback. Keeping the stool soft and bulky so it's easy for weakened muscles to expel is ideal. But if it's too soft it can become pasty and even more difficult to get out, and if it's too loose it can leak out.

ANATOMICAL CONSIDERATIONS

As I've mentioned, women have a naturally more convoluted colon, thanks to an extra ten centimeters (four inches) in length to allow for increased absorption during pregnancy. Women also have a wider gynecoid pelvis, which means that the female colon tends to drop down into the deeper pelvis, where it has to share space with the uterus, bladder, ovaries, and Fallopian tubes. Things tend to get all bunched up in this relatively small space. In men the colon is less likely to drop down into the narrower android pelvis, and most of the male colon is located in the roomier abdomen. These anatomical differences explain why women are disproportionately more constipated and bloated. It also explains why colonoscopy in women frequently takes twice as long and requires more sedation.

Women can also develop fibroids, cysts, and endometriosis in the pelvis, which can press on the colon, causing bloating, constipation, and even a partial bowel obstruction. Scar tissue in the abdomen or pelvis from previous surgery or radiation can have the same effect.

SLOW TRANSIT/COLONIC INERTIA/DYSMOTILITY

Slow transit through the colon backs things up, but this time the stool isn't all clustered at the back door waiting to come out; it's spread out throughout the colon. Dietary factors like not consuming enough fiber and water are huge causes of slow transit, but so are medications that slow down peristalsis, including narcotic pain medications, antidepressants, vitamins that contain iron, calcium channel blockers, and aluminum-containing antacids. It's a long list, so the medicine cabinet is always a good place to look if you have slow transit.

Hormonal changes, especially around menopause, and systemic conditions like an underactive thyroid that slow everything down also contribute to slow transit. Diabetes can affect the nerves that control gut motility and result in things either moving too fast (diarrhea) or too slow (constipation). Long-term laxative use, particularly of stimulant laxatives, can lead to colonic inertia where the bowels becomes less responsive and require increasing doses of laxative for defecation to occur.

The best way to diagnose this is a simple test called a Sitz marker study. You swallow a capsule containing about two dozen tiny rings. A few days later an X-ray of the abdomen is taken to show the position of the rings. Normally the majority of the rings (80 percent) will have been excreted. With obstructed defecation from anismus they'll often be clustered at the end of the colon, but with slow transit/colonic inertia/dysmotility, they'll be scattered throughout the colon.

DIET

As a society, we tend to be overfed but undernourished: 51 percent of the standard American diet consists of refined and processed foods, 42 percent is dairy and animal products, and only 7 percent comes from fiber-containing fruits and vegetables. We consume only a fraction of the recommended grams of daily fiber, and we pay for it in the bathroom with hard, small, and difficult-to-pass stools. Lots of patients tell me they eat tons of fiber, but they're referring to things like iceberg lettuce in salad and processed fiber in cereal that don't do much for bulking your stool and are of dubious nutritional value. Vegetables, legumes, and most fruits are filled with fiber and other nutrients and are key ingredients for improving constipation.

We know dairy can cause gas, bloating, and diarrhea in people who are lactose intolerant, but it can also cause constipation. Diets high in cheese and other low-fiber/high-fat foods like meat take longer to digest and can slow down motility. In addition, they tend to leave less room on your plate for the high-fiber grains and vegetables that relieve constipation.

SEDENTARY LIFESTYLE

A sedentary lifestyle can be a major contributor to slow transit through the GI tract, making constipation widely prevalent in places like nursing homes where the residents get little or no exercise. Exercise stimulates peristalsis and is an important tool in combating chronic constipation. As I'm fond of saying: if you're not moving, neither are your bowels!

DEPRESSION

Not only can depression itself lead to constipation, but many of the antidepressant drugs on the market are also associated with constipation. Opting for "talk therapy" over medication when appropriate and getting regular vigorous exercise may help treat both the depression and the constipation.

STRESS

Stress can worsen virtually every digestive condition, and constipation is no exception. Stress can disrupt the normal hormonal messages throughout the gut that are important for bowel regularity, as well as trigger the fight-or-flight response that diverts resources away from the digestive tract and suppresses the urge to evacuate.

Being in unfamiliar surroundings or disrupting your normal routine with travel will often result in constipation due to a change in diet, anxiety over using unfamiliar bathroom facilities, jet lag, and dehydration.

HORMONAL CHANGES

Many women report a change in bowel habits before their period, with a worsening of constipation as well as bloating and water retention. Menopause conspires to expand our waistline, increase water retention and gas, and slow down bowel activity, making us more constipated and bloated. That's because of fluctuating hormone levels and a phenomenon called estrogen dominance, which begins several years before we actually stop menstruating. An underactive thyroid gland, which can be subclinical and not detected by standard blood tests, is another common cause of constipation.

PREGNANCY

There are multiple causes of constipation during pregnancy, including: rising progesterone levels that relax smooth muscle and may decrease motility; morning sickness resulting in nausea, vomiting, and dehydration; the pressure of the expanding uterus on the rectum; prenatal vitamins that may contain iron and calcium; and a decrease in activity level. The combination of constipation and straining plus pressure from the uterus often results in hemorrhoids. A high-fiber diet, staying well hydrated, and maintaining some degree of physical activity are essential for maintaining regular bowel function during pregnancy.

DIVERTICULOSIS

The presence of small pockets in the colon that can fill with stool— otherwise known as diverticulosis (see Chapter 16)—is one of the commonest causes of a change in bowel habits in people over fifty. Often there are multiple small, incomplete bowel movements that are difficult to expel, so although there may be frequent passage, there is usually a feeling of constipation and bloating from stool being stuck and incomplete evacuation.

BACTERIAL IMBALANCE

Dysbiosis—a state of bacterial imbalance where there is overgrowth of harmful species and underrepresentation of "good bacteria" (see Chapter 6)—is a major cause of both constipation and bloating. Frequent antibiotics that kill off essential bacteria, medications that change the pH of the stomach and make it more hospitable to invading bacteria, and a diet high in sugar and fat are common causes of dysbiosis, which can also manifest as loose stool in some people.

GLUTEN INTOLERANCE/CELIAC DISEASE

Almost 1 percent of the population in America has celiac disease (see Chapter 11), and millions more are intolerant of gluten, the protein found in wheat, rye, and barley. Although celiac disease was originally thought of as a wasting illness with diarrhea and weight loss caused by malabsorption, these days constipation, bloating, and weight gain are among the most common symptoms, partly because gluten-containing grains themselves can be constipating, even in the absence of celiac disease or gluten intolerance. The weight gain happens because wheat products release a tremendous amount of glucose into the bloodstream when digested.

IRRITABLE BOWEL SYNDROME

Irritable bowel syndrome (IBS) (see Chapter 13) is a common cause of constipation that itself can have many causes, from undiagnosed celiac disease to candida overgrowth. Along with initiating therapy, investigating the underlying cause of the constipation is an important part of getting the symptoms under control.

NEUROLOGICAL CONDITIONS

Some of the most constipated patients I see suffer from multiple sclerosis (MS). The signals to the brain that are involved in defecation can get disrupted in MS, interfering with muscular relaxation. Pelvic floor disorders also frequently occur and bowel incontinence can be a problem, although constipation is more common. One of my patients with MS has to digitate with every bowel movement—she inserts a finger into her vagina and presses on the puborectalis muscle to straighten the angle and facilitate emptying. Despite massive amounts of laxatives and fiber, that's the only way she's been able to move her bowels, although we're slowly having some success retraining her muscles using a combination of bio-feedback and electrical stimulation to achieve muscular relaxation. Spinal cord injuries, strokes, and Parkinson's can all cause debilitating consti-pation.

CANCER

Most causes of constipation are benign, but mechanical compression from cancerous tumors, particularly colon, uterine, and ovarian cancer, can obstruct the bowel and lead to severe constipation. Often there are accom-panying symptoms like weight loss, blood in the stool, and vaginal bleed-ing, but sometimes bloating and a change in bowel habits with the new onset of constipation are the only initial signs.

Gutbliss Solutions for Constipation

Since constipation is a symptom, not a disease, it's always important to get to the root of what's causing the slowdown. It may be multiple things—for example, diet, lack of exercise, medications, and fibroids—so you may need multiple solutions. Here are some of my favorites, many of which are de-tailed in the 10-Day Gutbliss Plan (see Chapter 23):

Consider a Fiber Supplement

Creating a bigger, bulkier stool with fiber can lead to more effective triggering of the stretch receptors in the rectum, which can be very helpful if you're con-stipated. Keep in mind that if you have anismus, fiber alone might not be a remedy because it doesn't fix the relaxation problem. But lots of people have a mixed picture with an element of anismus and also not enough fiber, so it's worth trying a fiber supplement and also increasing the fiber in your diet.

I recommend using ground psyllium husk and starting slowly. Psyllium is a type of soluble plant fiber that doesn't get digested and helps to create a larger, bulkier stool that is easier to expel. Think of it like a broom that sweeps debris out of your colon and keeps the products of digestion moving through efficiently. Even if you follow a high-fiber diet, you can still benefit from the additional fiber in psyllium.

Too large a dose of psyllium at one time can clog up the bowels and worsen symptoms. Drinking it with a lot of water is essential to prevent it from clumping in the intestines.

Here's what I recommend, to start:

- 1 teaspoon of finely ground psyllium husk once a day in the morning, mixed with at least 8 ounces of liquid and followed by an additional 8-ounce glass of water.

You may feel full and even more bloated the first few days, but after a week your body should be used to the increased fiber. Then:

- After a week, add a second teaspoon in the middle of the day.
- After two weeks, add a third teaspoon at bedtime.
- Be sure to follow each dose with an additional glass of water.

What brand of psyllium should you buy? The kind that tastes good enough that you'll use it regularly. My hard-core patients like pure ground psyllium husk without any flavoring or additives. The particles are a little bigger, it has a kind of birdseed consistency, and it doesn't dissolve that well, but it has a very robust effect on the bowels. A more finely ground, smoother-texture, flavored psyllium is what a lot of other patients use. It dissolves more easily and tastes pretty good, although I'm not a fan of the artificially sweetened versions or the kind with lots of other additives.

If you're going to mix psyllium with something other than water, consider adding a little splash of juice or lemonade, but don't use too much juice or it will be too thick.

Also, you need to drink it briskly. If you sip it slowly, it tends to congeal and is hard to get down.

If you're constipated and also trying to lose a few pounds, a dose of ground psyllium husk three times a day will keep you full in between meals and is a healthy way to curb your appetite and treat your constipation at the same time.

Drink More Water

Much of your body (and a lot of your stool) consists of water. Drinking more of it is a simple step that can have significant results. The thirst mechanism that sends you in search of hydration doesn't kick in until you're already pretty dehydrated, and by then it can be hard to catch up, so measuring the amount of water you're drinking is really important.

The exact amount you need will depend on your size, your energy expenditure, how much you get from other sources like fruits and vegetables, what medications you take, what climate you live in, and whether or not you consume other liquids like soda, coffee, or caffeinated tea that can have a diuretic effect and actually dehydrate you. My recommendation is at least a liter of water a day. Start with that and increase it if it doesn't seem like enough or if you live in a hot climate.

Examining your urine will also help you to assess whether you're getting enough water. Ideally you should be urinating about four to seven times a day, and the color should be a pale yellow, although certain vitamins and medications can give it a more concentrated yellow color.

Move

Regular exercise is important to stimulate peristalsis and keep the products of digestion moving efficiently through your digestive tract. You don't have to run a marathon; even a walk around the block can help. I'm particularly fond of twisting yoga poses for helping disperse gas pockets and moving things along. See Chapter 21, "On the Move Toward Gutbliss," for more on how exercise stimulates the gut and improves bloating and constipation.

Clean Out the Medicine Cabinet

Many different medications, both prescription and over-the-counter, can cause or contribute to constipation and bloating. Some of the common ones include antidepressants, painkillers, blood pressure medications, vitamins with iron, and antacids. It's worth looking through your medicine cabinet and checking to see if something you're taking on a regular basis may be constipating you. Ask your doctor or pharmacist if you're not sure.

Develop Good Bathroom Habits

Every time you ignore the urge to go, you're training your digestive tract to be unresponsive. I see people with this sort of bowel confusion every day who literally don't know whether their stool is coming or going. Settling in with the newspaper, getting on a conference call, or delving into a good book when you're on the toilet are additional behaviors that untrain your bowels. They send a clear message to your brain and body that you have all day, encouraging sluggish bowel emptying.

Bowel training for those with erratic bowel movements involves sitting on the toilet at approximately the same time every morning to encourage a Pavlovian-type response. Your colon and pelvic muscles eventually get the message that sitting on the toilet means action.

Getting in and out efficiently is equally important. The best stoolers are as precise as a Swiss watch. My father, who is an Olympic contender for regularity, has a bowel movement at six a.m. every morning, regardless of where he is, what time he went to bed, or what he had for dinner. My mother, who is erratic with both her bathroom visits and her fiber supplement, can go days with no action and never knows where or when her next bowel movement may appear.

Create the Right Environment

I can and will use the bathroom anywhere, although at home, my preference is the master bathroom upstairs. The half bathroom downstairs seems a bit exposed and more public since it opens onto the living room and has a large window that faces our neighbor's patio. To get to the master bathroom, you have to walk through our closet, which adds a tucked-away feeling that makes it seem more private and less susceptible to interruption. There's a small window looking out onto the street, but the blinds are always drawn and the lighting is soft, adding to the coziness and warmth of the space. Creating the right ambience in your bathroom is essential for having good bowel movements. Temperature, lighting, accessibility, and privacy—all are important. Think of it as part of caring for and tending to your body, just like taking a warm bath to relax your muscles, applying lotion to moisturize and soothe, and doing all the other personal things that happen in the bathroom.

Change Your Position

Most people don't realize that their position when having a bowel movement is also key. Squatting is the most natural stance for giving birth and, it turns out, for having a bowel movement, too. A squatting position helps to straighten the anorectal angle and keeps the knees pressed up against the abdomen, increasing intra-abdominal pressure, which helps to push the stool out. Over a billion people throughout the world don't have access to toilets and squat over a hole instead. Interestingly, people in countries where squatting is the norm have much less constipation and colon cancer, probably because their diets, like their bathrooms, are less refined.

I'm not suggesting that you get rid of your modern plumbing, but sometimes getting back to nature isn't such a bad thing. The Squatty Potty is a small bench that you put your feet on to draw your legs up and closer to your chest when sitting on the toilet. It lets you approximate a squatting position while maintaining the luxury of a toilet rather than a hole in the ground. Putting your feet on a stack of phone books (or, no pun intended, a low stool) can achieve the same effect. If you're flexible, drawing your feet up and placing them on the toilet seat works great, too—but be careful not to fall off! I find that constipation is rarely entirely due to position, but every little bit counts in our quest for stool nirvana, so consider trying a squat to see if it helps.

Try Biofeedback

One of the most useful strategies for treating constipation, pelvic floor disorders, and anismus is biofeedback. Biofeedback is the process of getting your mind and body in sync. Anorectal biofeedback employs an internal sensor placed in the anal canal that records the pressure generated by the pelvic floor muscles. The readings are visually displayed to the patient via a monitor, and over time, the muscles are trained to respond in a more coordinated manner. (Biofeedback can be used for lots of things, not just constipation, and the types of sensors employed vary depending on the condition. For migraines, sensors that detect brain wave activity are used).

General biofeedback, without an internal sensor, is also helpful for constipation. A belly belt is worn around the waist that measures respiration, and sensors on the fingers measure temperature, heart rate, and blood flow.

The biofeedback practitioner first gets baseline or resting measurements. Then he or she will ask you to think about something stressful to see how your measurements change.

Then the real work begins. You'll be coached in using visual imagery, guided meditation, deep breathing, and other relaxation techniques to achieve a relaxed state where the indicators start to sync up, particularly the breath and the heart rate, and the muscles start to relax.

Although some people require more sessions than others, biofeedback has been an extraordinarily useful part of my practice. It's extremely helpful for you to see your heart rate decrease or your temperature warm as your blood vessels relax and dilate. You see the changes on the computer at the same time as you feel the effects in your body. The goal is that after a few sessions you're able to achieve the results on your own without the use of sensors or a computer.

Turn Around and Take a Look

Debunking the notion of stool and the bowels as being dirty is an important part of developing good bowel habits. A bowel movement isn't something shameful that should be furtive and secretive. I encourage my eight-year-old to look at her stool and to explore the connection between what she eats and drinks and how her stool looks and feels. When she complains of chalky pebbles that are hard to come out, she knows she has to eat more green vegetables or beans and drink a few more glasses of water. We've oohed and aahed together over some of her impressive stools the day after a big bowl of lentil soup. She knows what she has to do, even though she isn't always excited about doing it, and she'd still rather eat cookies than kale.

Making these connections between how she's living and how she's feeling is a crucial part of my daughter's education and her ability to care for herself as she gets older. I want her to know, not just intellectually but to feel in her physical body, the results she can create by making healthy choices. And I want the same thing for you.

PART 2

What's Gone Wrong in Your Gut?

5

Could It Be the Air You Swallow and the Gas You Pass?

THE QUESTION OF WHETHER TO CALL THE UPWARD EXPULSION OF AIR from the digestive tract through the mouth a burp or a belch seems to me to be one of pressure. Loud and aggressive passage sounds more like a belch; it has that frat-boy, stale-beer feeling. A burp, on the other hand, makes me think of something small and quiet that could go undetected behind a hand-embroidered handkerchief.

What about gas from below? The term *flatulence* derives from the Latin *flatus*—a blowing or breaking of wind, which connotes gentle breezes and may not capture the reality of dealing with daily gas and bloating. *Fart* may more precisely describe it, and although it's one of the oldest words in the English language, the fact that it made comedian George Carlin's original seven-dirty-words list speaks volumes.

All humor aside, the fact is that burping, belching, flatulence, and farting are normal bodily functions, but when they happen in excess, they can signal something amiss in your digestive tract. In this chapter I'll tell you about a common but frequently unrecognized condition that causes lots of burping, belching, and bloating. We'll also explore the mysteries of what causes gas, foods commonly associated with it, and some practical recommendations for how to generate less of it.

Swallowing Air

Aerophagia is a condition in which people swallow large amounts of air unintentionally and without realizing it. It's an incredibly common cause of bloating that can be misdiagnosed as acid reflux, ulcers, gallstones, or bacterial overgrowth.

Most of us swallow a bit of air when we eat or drink, and we may take in extra gas bubbles with carbonated beverages like seltzer, beer, soda, or champagne. But people with aerophagia swallow large amounts of air that can lead to a significant buildup of gas in their GI tract and, hence, major bloating.

If you have chronic sinus problems, a deviated septum, or a history of allergies or asthma, you may be prone to aerophagia because you frequently engage in mouth breathing, which predisposes you to air swallowing. Chewing gum, sucking on hard candy, smoking, eating too quickly, talking while eating, drinking liquids with meals, or wearing loose dentures can all cause aerophagia.

Most people with aerophagia come in complaining of three things: bloating, burping, and abdominal discomfort. Your stomach may feel tight like a drum and very distended because of the high pressure caused by all the swallowed air in there. I've had patients say they wish I could stick them with a pin to deflate them. Eventually most of the air gets burped up or makes its way through your GI tract and exits through the other end, but not without causing a lot of discomfort in between.

Some people with aerophagia swallow small amounts of air and force up burps repetitively as part of an anxiety syndrome. It's a nervous habit, like biting your fingernails or playing with your hair, and although it's a voluntary action, the person is usually unaware that he or she is doing it. One of my patients burped repetitively every ten or twenty seconds, but when I distracted her, it stopped completely. Biofeedback using deep breathing techniques and visualization to induce a more relaxed state eventually improved her burping. She still burps a lot when she's really nervous, but she's much more aware of it and now has the tools to control it.

One of my favorite aerophagia patients left me a five-minute voice mail of his burps. He was a pastor and extremely inconvenienced and embarrassed by his pathological burping, and he wanted to impress upon me how much of a problem it was. After listening to the voice mail, I was duly impressed. His situation was so severe that I immediately called in my colleague Susan Miller, PhD, who's an expert at diagnosing and treating aerophagia.

Susan carefully evaluated the pastor, analyzing his breathing, speaking, eating, and drinking patterns. She discovered that an undiagnosed deviated septum was causing him to breathe almost exclusively through his mouth. Breath holding was also a contributing factor—during his sermons he would speak loudly for long periods of time without breathing, then gasp for air in between sentences. Much of that air was being swallowed and by the end of the sermon he was looking and feeling like the Michelin man. Septoplasty surgery to fix his septum and retraining of his speech and breathing patterns put an end to his aerophagia and bloating.

If you suffer from aerophagia, chances are you've tried taking an antacid, which probably didn't help much, because although acid can enter the esophagus during a burp, aerophagia is caused by air, not acid.

Chew on This

People with aerophagia aren't the only ones who burp a lot. Commercially farmed cows each burp up over two hundred liters of methane gas a day. If you think that sounds like a lot, it is. Ten cows could produce enough methane gas to heat a small house for a year! They're a larger contributor to the greenhouse effect than coal mines, landfills, and sewage treatment plants.

Cows are ruminants, which means that their digestion begins with softening the food in the first part of their stomach to form what's called cud. They then regurgitate the partially digested cud into their mouth and chew it again. Rumination predisposes a body to burping because a certain amount of gas is emitted during regurgitation. However, if you take the average domesticated cow eating genetically engineered corn and soy on the feed lot and feed them grass instead, their gut bacteria changes and they produce much less gas.

Cows are meant to roam around and eat grass, and when they do, their GI tracts are much happier and they burp up less gas. Similarly, gas in

Gutbliss Solutions for Aerophagia

If you're bloated and think you may have aerophagia, try these tips:

- Spit out the gum.
- Don't suck on hard candy.
- Eat slowly.
- Don't talk on the phone while eating.
- Save drinking liquids for the beginning or end of the meal. Drink flat, not bubbly.
- Meditate a little if you feel anxious.
- Practice taking deep breaths that expand your lungs not your stomach.

If you're still not getting anywhere, a speech pathologist may help you identify if the problem is related to your respiratory, speech, or swallowing patterns.

humans, whether from above or below, can be a sign of an unhappy GI tract and a clue that you may be eating or drinking something that your intestines are having trouble digesting.

Bad Gas

Bad gas represents feedback from your digestive system that it doesn't like what you're putting in it. Let's look at some of the most common culprits.

LACTOSE

Lactose intolerance is a good example of bad gas. Many of us lose our ability to digest dairy products as we age. In fact, more than half the world's population has some degree of lactose intolerance, where the small intestine doesn't make enough of the enzyme lactase necessary for digesting the lactose sugar in milk. Gas and bloating are classic symptoms of lactose intolerance, but it can be tricky to diagnose because the symptoms overlap with so many other conditions, including irritable bowel syndrome (IBS), celiac disease, *Helicobacter pylori* infection, and gallstones.

Good Gas and Bad Gas

All gas is not created equal. Beans and cruciferous vegetables like cabbage, cauliflower, kale, and broccoli contain potent cancer-fighting compounds and lots of healthy fiber, but they also contain an indigestible sugar called raffinose. Bacteria in the colon ferment raffinose and produce methane, which you may experience as smelly gas. That's what I consider good gas, because it's accompanied by the health benefits that eating those foods confers.

If you think you may be lactose intolerant but you're not sure, try avoiding any and all dairy for a minimum of two weeks to see if your symptoms improve. You can also do more formal testing involving breath or blood tests. If you're missing the enzyme lactase, then a test dose of lactose will pass undigested into your colon, where it will be fermented by bacteria into hydrogen that can be detected in a breath test. A blood test that measures the amount of glucose in your blood after drinking a lactose solution is another way to check for lactose intolerance. Failure of your blood sugar to rise indicates your body isn't adequately digesting and absorbing lactose.

Once the diagnosis of lactose intolerance is made, either by evaluating the effects of removing dairy from your diet or with a test, then eliminating dairy products is a perfectly reasonable way to control your bloating. Most people have varying degrees of lactose intolerance and can tolerate small amounts of dairy but will have symptoms with larger doses. If your symptoms are mild and you can't live without some dairy, I recommend sticking to small amounts of yogurt and a little hard cheese, which contain less lactose than foods like ice cream, milk, and mozzarella.

Lactose intolerance is exceedingly common, but it can also be a sign of other problems in the GI tract. Celiac disease and Crohn's disease both affect the lining of the small intestine and can cause secondary lactose intolerance. Gastrointestinal infections like giardia and rotavirus are also common causes of lactose intolerance, which can end up being temporary or permanent.

If you're bloated, irrespective of whether or not you have lactose intol-

Gutbliss Solutions for Good Gas

I never recommend avoiding the "good gas" foods altogether because they contain lots of nutrients. Here are some things you can do to cut down on the gas when eating them:

If you haven't been eating foods like broccoli, kale, and cauliflower, start with a small amount and gradually increase your serving size to let your body get acclimated to them.

Add lemon juice to your good-gas veggies to stimulate digestive enzymes.

Soak beans overnight before cooking.

Avoid canned beans, which not only tend to cause more gas but may also contain a chemical called bisphenol A (BPA) in the can lining, which has been linked to cancer and other conditions.

Cook beans with a sea vegetable like kombu, which makes the beans more digestible because it contains the enzyme needed to break down raffinose. You can find kombu at Asian markets or health food stores.

Take Beano or Bean-zyme at the start of a meal. Like kombu, these products contain a plant-derived enzyme that breaks down raffinose.

Eat a pinch (about ⅛ teaspoon) of fennel seeds or chew on a stalk of raw fennel at the end of a meal to benefit from its gas-reducing oils. You can also make fennel tea by steeping a teaspoon of crushed seeds or fresh fennel bulbs in a cup of boiling water for 10 minutes, or you can add it to salads or cooked dishes.

Boost your GI tract's population of "good" bacteria by consuming fermented foods like kefir and sauerkraut that contain actively growing essential bacteria and helpful yeast species that result in decreased gas production.

erance, you may find that eliminating or cutting back on your dairy intake improves your symptoms. Since there's no compelling reason to consume dairy—you can get lots of calcium from green vegetables, beans, sesame seeds, and fish, and weight-bearing exercise is a great way to prevent osteoporosis—you don't have anything to lose, except possibly your bloat.

FRUCTOSE

Lactose isn't the only sugar that could be causing your bloating. Fructose malabsorption affects 30 percent of the population and is frequently misdiagnosed as IBS. Fructose occurs naturally in fresh fruit and some vegetables and is present in high amounts in dried or canned fruit and fruit juices. But the main source of fructose in the American diet is high fructose corn syrup added to sweeten products like soda, cereals, desserts, candy, salad dressing, ketchup, and most packaged foods.

Normally a person can absorb about 25 to 50 grams of fructose per day, but people with fructose malabsorption absorb much less, and current research suggests an increased risk for medical conditions such as osteoporosis, elevated triglycerides, heart disease, and inflammation with more than 50 grams of fructose a day. A can of regular soda has about 23 grams of fructose, and the Standard American Diet can lead to consumption of hundreds of grams of fructose per day. Bacteria in the colon break the excess unabsorbed fructose down into short-chain fatty acids. The by-products include lots of hydrogen, methane, and carbon dioxide gas, along with weight gain and diabetes.

LOW-CALORIE SWEETENERS

When it comes to food, it's helpful to remember that you can't get something for nothing. In the case of sweeteners, your choices are calories or gas. Many low-calorie sweeteners are made of sugar alcohols called polyols and include sorbitol, mannitol, erythritol, and xylitol. They're used to sweeten candy and chocolates marketed to diabetics, and if you've ever eaten them, you know they can cause impressive bloating and gas. These substances are incompletely absorbed in the small intestine, which is why they contribute little in the way of calories, but they're fermented in the colon by bacteria, where they contribute a lot in the way of gas.

Sugar alcohols definitely count as a cause of bad gas in my book. You're much better off having a little sugar from time to time than subjecting your intestines to this kind of discomfort.

If you think your bloating may be a result of lactose, fructose, or sugar alcohol malabsorption, you may consider trying the FODMAPS diet that minimizes carbohydrates that can be poorly absorbed in some people.

Gutbliss Solutions for Bad Gas

Identifying and reducing potential sources of bad gas can help you banish your bloat. Here are some suggestions:

Eliminate dairy for a couple of weeks to see if you may be lactose intolerant, or consider a breath or blood test to confirm the diagnosis.

If you're lactose intolerant, you may still be able to tolerate small amounts of hard cheese and yogurt, which contain less lactose than soft cheeses and milk.

Avoid high fructose corn syrup, to ensure you're within the daily limit of fructose absorption of about 50 grams.

If you think you might be one of the 30 percent of the population that have fructose malabsorption, you may only be able to tolerate half the recommended limit (25 grams).

Choose more natural sources of fructose, such as fresh fruits and vegetables, over the fructose in processed food and soda.

Pay attention to unexpected sources of fructose, such as applesauce, dried fruits, cereal, fruit juices, and salad dressings.

Choose calories over gas when it comes to sweeteners. Low-calorie sweeteners made of sugar alcohols aren't absorbed in the small intestine and produce a lot of gas when they undergo additional fermentation by bacteria in the colon.

Cut down on sulfur-rich foods like eggs, meat, yogurt, and seafood.

Consider trying the FODMAPs diet, which minimizes poorly absorbed short-chain carbohydrates, including most dairy, corn syrup, wheat products, certain vegetables, and fruit with a high glucose-to-fructose ratio, such as watermelon and dried fruit.

FODMAPS stands for fermentable oligosaccharides, disaccharides, monosaccharides, and polyols. It was developed by Australian researchers as a way to reduce IBS symptoms with the theory being that eating low FODMAP foods reduces hydrogen and methane production and improves gas, bloating, and abdominal pain. The diet restricts most dairy, corn syrup, wheat products, certain vegetables, and fruit with a high glucose-to-fructose ratio like watermelon and dried fruit. Although you don't necessarily need to be as strict as the researchers were in their original study, following a low FODMAPs diet may help get your gas and bloating under control.

The Gas You Pass

Everyone has gas, which we either burp up or expel through our rectum. Undoubtedly, some of us have more than others. On average we produce over a liter of gas a day and, whether we acknowledge it or not, pass gas about a dozen times. The gas we pass consists primarily of the breakdown of undigested material by bacteria in the colon, which produces mostly odorless gases like oxygen, carbon dioxide, nitrogen, hydrogen, and methane, plus a contribution from swallowed air.

Smelly gas is usually a result of additional fermentation by bacteria in the colon, particularly when you're eating sulfur-rich foods like eggs, meat, dairy, and cruciferous vegetables that can produce smelly hydrogen sulfide gas. The particular mix of bacterial species in your colon will also influence the odor of your gas. Excessive or foul-smelling gas from above or below doesn't necessarily mean something's wrong in your GI tract, but it can be a sign that you're ingesting something that doesn't agree with you, and it might be worthwhile experimenting with decreasing or eliminating some of the foods I've discussed in this chapter. As far as I know, no one has ever died from passing gas, but optimizing the air you swallow and the gas you pass can lead to significant improvements in your bloating and your quality of life.

Trouble in the Microbiome?

THERE ARE MORE THAN ONE BILLION BACTERIA IN EACH DROP OF FLUID in your colon, an environment we call the microbiome. It's a mixture so distinctive from person to person that your individual constellation of bacteria is a more specific identifier than your own DNA. Your unique bacterial footprint develops over your lifetime, and it reflects what you've eaten, where you've lived, past infections, exposure to chemicals, hormone levels, antibiotics and other medications you've taken, and even your emotions—stress can have a profound effect on gut bacteria. A balanced mix with a much higher ratio of "good" or beneficial to "bad" or potentially harmful species is crucial for effective digestion.

The solid matter in bowel movements consists of about 50 percent bacteria, and which particular species are present in your stool and your gut is an important determinant of whether you'll end up bloated or not. But imbalance in your gut bacteria doesn't just cause bloating; it can lead to lots of other serious medical problems. In this chapter we'll explore the factors that can adversely affect the delicate ecosystem within your intestines and talk about how to restore your gut bacteria, or flora, to a state of balance and bliss.

Antibiotics: Friend or Foe?

I'm going to tell you a story about the love of my life—my daughter, Sydney Kamala. Because she was only born in 2005, it's not a long story, but there are aspects of it I wish I could rewrite, and as a mother and a physician, I feel a strong calling to share what I learned. Fortunately, it doesn't have a sad ending, but it's a story I see repeated over and over. Not only can what happened to Sydney lead to really bad bloating and digestive upset down the road, but it's also associated with more serious problems like autoimmune disorders.

My labor started at eight a.m. and ended abruptly just after midnight. I had thought Sydney would pop out easily, but hours passed and still no baby. The ubiquitous "failure to progress" during labor prompted a C-section, which I dreaded and had tried my best to avoid. The rate of C-sections in the United States is now one in three births, and while many are medically necessary, as I assume mine was, a huge number are based on convenience and the widespread use of labor-inducing drugs like oxytocin, which I had also received.

C-sections bypass a critical early step in the maturation of a child's immune system: colonization with the mother's vaginal bacteria. A study published in the *Proceedings of the National Academy of Sciences* in 2010 shows that babies born vaginally are colonized with more *Lactobacillus* species and other "good bacteria," whereas C-section babies tend to be colonized with more common hospital "bad bacteria," such as *Staphylococcus*. Swallowing a mouthful of microbes as you pass through the birth canal confers important benefits in later life, including a lower likelihood of developing asthma, allergies, and other immune-related diseases.

In addition to missing out on those early essential bugs, Sydney received two strong intravenous antibiotics immediately after delivery. I'd had the flu and a fever when I went into labor, so despite her being healthy with no evidence of infection, it was decided to treat her as if she had one. At the time I thought it was great that the doctors were being so proactive and giving my healthy newborn antibiotics "just in case."

At about six months old, Sydney had her first ear infection. A high fever, vomiting, and inconsolable screaming led to the first of what would be many, many visits to the pediatrician. Over the next year and a half,

Sydney received over a dozen courses of antibiotics for fever, pharyngitis, and ear infections.

What concerned me the most was that no one really seemed to be paying attention to how many rounds of antibiotics she'd received. The doctor would look at the last page of her chart, see what antibiotic she had last been on, and prescribe something similar. Every few months we graduated to a more potent antibiotic as the critters making her sick became increasingly resistant. I didn't want to be *that* kind of patient: the kind who asks pointed, uncomfortable questions—such as whether a dozen rounds of antibiotics in a young child are really necessary or a good idea, or what alternative solutions might exist. Philosophically, I hadn't yet had my awakening—I still wholeheartedly believed in the superiority of modern medicine, the omniscience of the doctor, and the seductive simplicity of "illness equals antibiotics."

But does it really?

- Studies show that 68 percent of patients seeking treatment for acute respiratory tract problems are prescribed antibiotics, which in 80 percent of cases are later found to be unnecessary based on Centers for Disease Control and Prevention (CDC) guidelines.
- A Harvard study of antibiotics for the treatment of sore throats in over four thousand children found that the rate of treatment greatly exceeded the rate of positive results and that actual testing for strep and other pathogens was only done in about half of the children who were prescribed antibiotics.
- In 2010 the *Journal of the American Medical Association* (*JAMA*) published a study that found that treating children with antibiotics for ear infections, which are mostly viral, did little to speed recovery and was associated with an increased risk of side effects, like rashes and diarrhea.

The Era of "Over" Everything

Alexander Fleming's discovery of penicillin in 1928 is still one of the greatest contributions to medicine. It could have prevented events like the Great Plague of the seventeenth century, which wiped out a quarter of the population of Europe. But now we've entered a different era: the era of overdiagnosis and overtreatment. It's estimated in the *International Journal of Microbial Agents* that 20 to 50 percent of all antibiotic use is inappropriate, resulting in an increased risk of side effects, higher costs (over $1 billion annually on unnecessary antibiotics for respiratory tract infections in adults alone!), and resistance to antibiotics. It's not a coincidence that flesh-eating strains of *Streptococcus* and refractory *Clostridium difficile*—infections previously seen primarily in sick hospitalized patients—are now widespread in the community, and that food allergies, bloating, and digestive upset have become ubiquitous. H. Gilbert Welch, MD, MPH, discusses the dangers of this type of medicine in his excellent book *Overdiagnosed: Making People Sick in the Pursuit of Health*.

While I never requested or pushed for antibiotics for Sydney, I didn't refuse them, either, and the cycle of prescriptions and illness continued, including a hospitalization for *Rotavirus* and prolonged antibiotics for nondraining fluid in her ear. And then something happened that really made me reconsider what I was subjecting my child to.

Sydney had had a cold and a lingering cough, so my husband took her to the doctor. They returned from the visit carrying a nebulizer machine for asthma and four prescriptions: steroids, antibiotics, antihistamines, and a bronchodilator!

I was shocked by the new diagnosis and the amount of medication. Sydney had never shown any signs of asthma. She had a cold and an accompanying cough, as did everyone in the family that winter. I took everything up to the attic and put it in a storage box. I pulled out the wad of pharmacy stubs and insurance receipts that I'd been diligently filing after every visit and started counting: fifteen courses of antibiotics; and between the pediatrician, allergist, and ear, nose, and throat specialist, over forty visits to the doctor—far more than I'd had in my entire life— and she hadn't even started kindergarten! That was when I decided it was time for a new approach: the less-is-more approach.

Aside from the annual pilgrimage to get her forms for school signed, we stopped going to the doctor. And something interesting happened; the fewer the visits and the antibiotics, the healthier Sydney became. Sydney's good bacteria had been so depleted from the barrage of antibiotics starting at birth that she had trouble fighting even a simple viral infection.

Initially she still developed a respiratory tract infection and fever almost every month, but eventually the frequency and severity of those episodes started to wane. Her immune system began to recover from the onslaught of antibiotics, and her overall resilience and health improved.

But the fallout wasn't all good. One of the most dramatic changes after Sydney was hospitalized for *Rotavirus* was her craving for sugar. As if someone had flipped a switch, suddenly she couldn't get enough of it. Our diet was quite balanced, and Sydney had previously been happily eating the same food we did without any complaints. When she was discharged from the hospital, I thought a sugar-craving alien had taken over my daughter's body. She woke up in the morning asking about dessert and went to bed strategizing about the next bowl of ice cream. At the time I was baffled and confused, but now I recognize that the cravings were due to overgrowth of yeast species, which thrive on sugar, and other changes in her gut flora from all the antibiotics. Although much improved, it's something we're still working on correcting.

In hindsight it seems so intuitive to me now that Sydney was overdiagnosed and overtreated, but I was a first-time mother trying hard not to second-guess the medical establishment that I myself was firmly entrenched in. I was in the same position so many of my patients find themselves in: relying on doctors who really are trying their best, as Sydney's doctors were, but whose practice is rooted in the narrow confines of conventional medicine with its overreliance on medications. I wish I had been wise enough to ask more questions and to say no more often—to do what I do now when Sydney has a cold: administer a home prescription of green veggie juice, homemade soup, and rest; get a swab for strep if she has a really bad sore throat; and avoid antibiotics unless we know what we're treating and she absolutely needs them, which she hasn't in years.

There are some infections that definitely require treatment, but more often the need for antibiotics is a gray zone, as demonstrated in a study published in the journal *Pediatrics* in which researchers examined the relationship between perceived expectation and pediatrician prescribing behavior. Astonishingly, they found that doctors prescribed antibiotics 62 percent of the time when they perceived parents expected them, and only 7 percent of the time when they thought parents didn't!

I realize that as a physician I have inside knowledge that makes it easier for me to decide whether a medication or a trip to the doctor is truly necessary, and in no way am I advocating that people stop taking their kids—or themselves—to the doctor when they're sick. But I am advocating that you become *that* kind of patient: the kind that asks questions about whether the antibiotic you've just been prescribed is really necessary or advisable, and what alternative solutions there might be, including watchful waiting and no medications.

The good news right now is that Sydney is a normal, healthy child. But I worry about autoimmune disease developing down the road; her history is so similar to many of my patients with Crohn's and ulcerative colitis who received lots of antibiotics at a young age when their immune system was still developing. My main weapon these days, in addition to avoiding unnecessary antibiotics, is steering her away from too much sugary, starchy food, and getting as many leafy greens into her as possible to encourage the growth of good bacteria. As we'll discover later in this chapter, we are what we eat when it comes to gut bacteria, and I believe that in the right setting, food can be potent medicine.

Are We Too Clean?

I'm seeing a virtual epidemic of bloating and digestive distress in people who have lots of symptoms but a normal-looking GI tract. The common thread in many of these patients is a history of frequent antibiotics. In fact, a detailed history of antibiotic use is one of the first things I ask about in new patients coming in to discuss their bloating. Some have a past similar to Sydney's: multiple antibiotics prescribed in childhood for pharyngitis or ear infections. Others took tetracycline or doxycycline as teenagers for months or even years for pimply skin. Some received antibiotics later in life for adult acne, recurrent sinus infections, or chronic Lyme disease.

I can't comment on how many of these antibiotics were truly necessary (your dermatologist is focused on solving your skin problems; GI distress isn't really on their radar), but I can tell you unequivocally that for many people, the bloating and GI upset they cause are devastating.

If we look at a map of the world, one of the striking observations is that inflammatory bowel diseases (Crohn's and ulcerative colitis), asthma, allergies, and autoimmune disorders like multiple sclerosis, lupus, and arthritis are common in more developed countries and rare in less developed ones. The so-called hygiene hypothesis explains this uneven distribution by suggesting that less childhood exposure to gut bacteria and parasites in affluent societies like the United States and Europe actually increases susceptibility to disease and allergies by suppressing the natural development of the immune system. It seems we need interaction with bugs to develop a strong immune system. People in poor countries are exposed to lots of different ones, and we now realize that this exposure may protect them from developing disease in later life. Not surprisingly, a diet high in fat and sugar is the other factor that correlates very strongly with the development of autoimmune diseases, since what we eat greatly determines what kinds of bacteria we develop.

We don't know specifically what causes illnesses like Crohn's and ulcerative colitis, but we do know that an immune system that hasn't been exposed to enough bacteria is strongly associated with disease, whether the bacteria have been wiped out by antibiotics, too many antibacterial cleaning products, a C-section, poor diet, an environment that's just too clean, or some combination of the above. What's become very clear, especially to people like me who specialize in autoimmune digestive diseases, is that bacteria aren't all bad, and, in fact, certain species are essential for digestive health.

Gut Bacteria: The Good, the Bad, and the Ugly

In order to understand how antibiotics wreak such havoc in the GI tract, we need to take a look at the role of gut bacteria. The trillions of microscopic organisms that make their home inside us can be categorized into three groups:

1. commensal or transitional flora, with whom we cohabit peacefully;
2. essential organisms, with whom we live symbiotically and whose existence benefits us; and
3. pathogens that can do us harm, often described as opportunistic flora or bad bacteria.

Bacteria are as integral to your body as the cells that make up your skin, bones, joints, brain, and other organs. In fact, the metabolic functions performed by your gut bacteria are as essential as those of many of your other organs. Microbial cells outnumber human cells ten to one, and the majority of them are in the gut, weighing a total of three to four pounds. Your specific and unique bacterial composition can affect lots of things: how you feel, how you look, your mood, your immunity to disease, and even your weight. We don't know exactly how many different bacterial species are represented in the gut, but estimates suggest five hundred to one thousand different types, plus viruses and fungi such as candida. And those are just the ones we know about.

Symbiotic organisms—the quintessential good bacteria—perform lots of important functions: they maintain a healthy immune system, keep our pH balanced, metabolize drugs and hormones, synthesize important nutrients and vitamins, neutralize cancer-causing compounds, and produce short-chain fatty acids (SCFAs) that provide intestinal cells with energy. Food can't be fully broken down and nutrients and vitamins can't be properly absorbed without adequate amounts of essential gut bacteria. This means that *even if you're eating a healthy diet, you may not be absorbing and assimilating the nutrients if your gut bacteria aren't optimized.* A well-functioning digestive system relies on the delicate balance between good and bad bacteria, without any one species becoming too over- or underrepresented.

When you take an antibiotic, you may experience nausea, diarrhea, or vomiting after just a couple of doses. But you may not realize that your long-term bloating could also be a direct result of antibiotics—those you took recently, as well as those from years or even *decades* ago. Antibiotics are supposed to kill pathogens, that is, bad bacteria, but they also indiscriminately kill off huge numbers of the good bacteria that are essential for a healthy gut. Unfriendly fungal species and other non-desirables quickly proliferate to fill the void created by the loss of good bacteria. Even previously benign commensals, if their numbers increase too much, can become problematic. The result is dysbiosis, a state of bacterial imbalance and one of the commonest causes of bloating and GI upset.

Dysbiosis isn't limited to the colon. Small intestinal bacterial overgrowth is a type of dysbiosis where an overabundance of bacteria develops in the small intestine, which normally contains much less bacteria than the colon. Dysbiosis can also occur on the skin or in the vagina, mouth, nose, sinuses, or ears. That's why, if you have bloating from bacterial imbalance, you may also have symptoms referable to these locations, including:

- Skin blemishes
- Vaginal discharge
- Burning sensation in the mouth
- Itchy ears
- Chronic sinus problems

Your doctor may have prescribed antibiotics for bacterial vaginosis (BV), cystic acne, or recurrent sinus infections, but that approach is often part of the problem, not the solution. Your vaginal discharge, blemishes, or sinuses may initially get better, but chances are you'll find yourself in a vicious cycle of recurring symptoms, and more antibiotics, as your bacterial balance is disrupted. Avoiding unnecessary antibiotics is essential not just for improving your bloating but for clearing up these other problems, too.

Some experts who study gut bacteria believe that dysbiosis contributes to many diseases, including autism, inflammation, depression, fibromyalgia, chronic fatigue syndrome, autoimmune disorders, cancer, and even obesity. Interestingly, lean people tend to be colonized with different bacterial species relative to their obese counterparts.

Yeast Overgrowth (Candida)

Fungal (yeast) overgrowth with organisms such as candida is a form of dysbiosis and something you may have experienced vaginally after taking antibiotics. Diabetics and immunocompromised individuals are particularly susceptible. Yeast proliferates in damp places, such as under your arms, in your groin, in your mouth, or in your rectum. Problems it can cause include:

- Nail infections
- Rectal itching
- Oral thrush (white lesions in the mouth)
- Skin problems such as eczema, acne, hives, athlete's foot, ringworm, and dandruff
- Fatigue
- Headaches
- Unstable blood sugar
- Food sensitivities
- Depression
- Impaired concentration

Yeast overgrowth in the body also causes bloating and gas, because yeast species are involved in the fermentation of food, a process that produces carbon dioxide gas. With overgrowth of yeast comes overproduction of carbon dioxide. An overabundance of yeast in the intestines can also be irritating to the lining, resulting in poor absorption of nutrients, and constipation or diarrhea.

Dysbiosis and Leaky Gut Syndrome

While dysbiosis definitely causes bloating, its association with what is known as leaky gut syndrome can be far more problematic. The inner lining of the intestines is a porous membrane, like a fishing net constructed of very fine mesh. Under normal circumstances, fat, protein, and carbohydrates are broken down, absorbed through the tiny holes in the membrane into the bloodstream, and transported to cells to be used for energy, cell division, and repair. The gut membrane also keeps threats to the body in the form of antigens, microbes, ingested chemicals, and toxic metabolic by-products from being absorbed through the net. Good stuff in, bad stuff out: that's how it's supposed to work. Unfortunately, the membrane is under constant attack, particularly when there's bacterial imbalance and overgrowth of potentially harmful microbes.

The number and type of bacteria in the digestive tract play a crucial role in maintaining the integrity of the membrane. With dysbiosis, particularly overgrowth of certain species like candida, the net can develop large holes. Substances that would normally have been kept in the gut and excreted in the stool instead pass through the membrane into the bloodstream. The immune system, sensing invaders, becomes roused, increasing the potential for autoimmune disease as the body starts to mount reactions to these foreign substances. Large, incompletely digested food particles may find their way into the bloodstream, resulting in multiple food sensitivities and allergies as the body doesn't fully recognize these unfamiliar substances and may treat them as enemies. On constant alert, the immune system can become very reactive, responding to all sorts of stimuli it would normally ignore. People with dysbiosis often complain of unusual reactions, including hives, rashes, itching, dizziness, and headaches. In addition to causing allergic reactions, these particles can find their way to other organs, causing inflammation and dysfunction.

Why Are Our Bacteria Out of Balance?

Why are our microbes so out of whack? There are a number of reasons, including the widespread use of antibiotics, not just those prescribed for humans but the large amounts given to some commercially raised animals that can end up in our food. The Western diet is another factor, as is the prevalence of acid-suppressing drugs and other medications that change the pH of the digestive tract and disrupt bacterial balance.

OVERTREATING WHAT WE EAT

A 2012 *New York Times* article shed some fascinating light on the use of antibiotics in the food industry. An astounding 80 percent of all antibiotics sold in the United States are used in animals raised for human consumption, either to treat infections (which can occur as a result of overcrowding) or to promote faster growth. The Food and Drug Administration (FDA) requires that milk contain no detectable antibiotics when tested, but random inspections have found dairy cows with illegal levels of antibiotics, raising concerns about the presence of antibiotics not just in meat but in the milk supply as well. These practices may contribute to the rise of widespread antibiotic resistance in humans.

OVEREATING THE WRONG FOODS

A sugary, starchy, fat-laden Western diet encourages growth of the wrong type of bacteria in your gut. Italian researchers compared children in Florence eating a typical Western diet with a group in a rural part of Africa eating fiber-rich legumes and vegetables. The gut bacteria were pretty similar in breastfed babies, but as children started to eat their local diet, the groups diverged significantly. The European group eating the high-fat/high-sugar diet had less microbial diversity and more species associated with diarrhea, allergy, and obesity. The African children had lots of species associated with leanness and also much higher levels of beneficial SCFAs known to protect against inflammation.

Too much sugar, fat, and processed carbohydrates can send bad bacteria into a feeding frenzy, leading to overgrowth. As I mentioned in the Introduction, that's what happened to me when I was overindulging in sugar-laden foods.

FORGETTING TO EAT FIBER

Not eating enough fiber encourages dysbiosis, too. Most Americans only eat about half the recommended 25 to 35 grams of fiber daily, which can negatively affect both the amount and diversity of bacterial species present. Certain types of dietary fiber are what we call prebiotics: non-digestible foods that encourage the growth of beneficial species and are a crucial part of restoring balance when dysbiosis is present. Studies have shown that eating soluble fiber from foods such as corn increases the population of helpful *Lactobacillus* species in the gut.

BLOCKING ACID

Many of us think of stomach acid only as something that makes us uncomfortable when it irritates our esophagus in acid reflux. But stomach acid is one of our main defenses against harmful bacteria that enter the body through the mouth. Drugs like proton pump inhibitors (PPIs) block acid so effectively that they can transform the stomach from an inhospitable site for invading bacteria into a friendly alkaline environment where bacteria can gain a foothold and multiply. Long-term PPI use may be a major factor in people with dysbiosis and bloating. By changing the pH of the intestines, these drugs don't just contribute to bacterial overgrowth; they are also associated with a decrease in the absorption of important nutrients such as iron, magnesium, vitamin B_{12}, and calcium and can increase your risk for developing fractures. Last but not least, the change in pH may render your digestive enzymes less effective, which adds to your bloat.

OTHER MEDICATIONS

Medications such as birth control pills, steroids, and chemotherapy can also cause or contribute to dysbiosis by altering your internal gut milieu. Fortunately, careful attention to your diet, maximizing your consumption of high-fiber fruits and vegetables, cutting down on caffeine and alcohol, decreasing your stress, and increasing your activity level can all help to combat the deleterious effects of these drugs.

Diagnosing and Treating Dysbiosis

The diagnosis of dysbiosis can be elusive—I find that breath and stool tests are only helpful about 50 percent of the time—and a close look at lifestyle habits and personal history is often the only way to make a good clinical diagnosis. Treatment, too, can be complex and highly individualized. I recommend a three-pronged approach that involves:

1. avoidance,
2. encouragement, and
3. repopulation.

AVOIDANCE

Avoid medications, foods, and other substances that contribute to the problem, including:

- Acid suppressors
- Alcohol
- Antacids
- Antibiotics
- Artificial sweeteners

- Birth control pills
- Hormone replacement therapy
- NSAIDs
- Steroids
- A sugary, starchy, fatty diet

Causes of Dysbiosis

Below is a list of some of the medications and conditions that can throw your beautiful intestinal balance seriously out of whack and cause dysbiosis:

- Acid suppressor drugs
- Alcohol
- Antibiotics
- Artificial sweeteners
- Birth control pills
- Bowel obstruction
- Chemotherapy
- Constipation
- Crohn's disease
- Decreased motility
- Diabetes
- Diverticulosis
- Fatty foods
- Fistulas
- Gastric bypass surgery
- Hormone therapy
- Hypochlorhydria (low acid)
- Hypothyroidism
- Immune deficiency
- Infections
- Low fiber
- Pancreatic enzyme deficiency
- Parasites
- Postoperative changes
- Scleroderma
- Steroids
- Stress
- Sugar overconsumption

ENCOURAGEMENT

Encourage the growth of good bacteria by consuming foods with prebiotic ingredients that stimulate the proliferation and activity of essential gut bacteria, including:

- Inulin, a naturally occurring carbohydrate that belongs to a class of dietary fibers called fructans. Inulin is found in plants like artichokes, chicory, and jicama.
- Oats, dandelion greens, garlic, leeks, onion, and asparagus, which also contain prebiotics, especially when consumed raw.
- Fermented foods, such as sauerkraut, cabbage, and kefir, which contribute to the growth of good bacteria, as do a wide variety of leafy green vegetables.

Stool as Medicine?

Clostridium difficile, also known as *C. diff*, is a bacterium associated with antibiotic use that can cause serious diarrheal illness and even death. When someone whose gut bacteria have been depleted from antibiotics encounters *C. diff* (often in a nursing home or hospital setting), it can proliferate in the gut, releasing toxins that cause severe diarrhea, cramping, bloating, and, in some cases, serious inflammation in the colon (pseudomembranous colitis).

   C. diff infection affects approximately 1 percent of all hospitalized patients in the United States, as a result of the widespread use of antibiotics—the main risk factor for acquiring the infection. Ironically, treatment with additional antibiotics has been the mainstay of therapy for *C. diff*, and perhaps not surprisingly, we're seeing a tremendous increase in the number of infections that are resistant to the standard antibiotic treatment.

   This has led to a novel new type of therapy: fecal transplants that involve transferring stool from healthy donors (usually a first-degree family member) into the digestive tract of the person infected with *C. diff*. The stool may be introduced in a number of ways: via a tube inserted through the nose that delivers it into the intestines; as a rectal enema; or placed in the colon during a colonoscopy. A study published by the *New England Journal of Medicine* showed that fecal transplants were far more effective in clearing up recurrent *C. diff* infection than standard antibiotic therapy, reinforcing the concept of how crucial our gut bacteria really are.

REPOPULATION

Repopulate the gut with large amounts of live bacteria in the form of a robust probiotic. Probiotics are live strains of bacteria that can be taken in pill, powder, or liquid form. They aren't considered drugs, so they're not regulated or tested for safety or efficacy, and sometimes marketing can masquerade as science on the various Internet sites that sell them. You may have to do some research to find out which particular type may be helpful for you.

   The two probiotics I use the most in my practice are VSL#3 and Align. VSL#3 is considered a medical food for certain conditions, including inflammatory bowel disease and irritable bowel syndrome. I also use it in people who've taken extensive antibiotics or had recent gastrointestinal infections. It contains massive amounts of bacteria, including three strains of *Bifidobacterium*, four strains of *Lactobacillus*, and one strain of *Streptococcus*, which help to crowd out pathogenic species and also produce nutrients necessary for proper function of the intestinal lining. Align contains *Bifidobacterium infantis* and works well for mild digestive upset.

You may experience worsened bloating after initially starting a probiotic as your bowels adjust to the increased bacterial load. While some people feel better after a week, others may need a month to notice significant improvement. A ninety-day course is often sufficient to repopulate the colon, while others may benefit from staying on a probiotic indefinitely, depending on their degree of bacterial imbalance and ongoing conditions that may be contributing to dysbiosis. Probiotics can make a big difference in your digestive wellness when used alongside other lifestyle changes. But relying on a probiotic alone to restore balance without considering the role of diet and lifestyle is sort of like eating at McDonald's every day and hoping a vitamin will provide you with whatever nutrients you might be missing. You have to really look at the big picture and all the contributing factors when it comes to your microbiome.

Identifying and remediating the cause of your bacterial imbalance is an essential step in the treatment of dysbiosis. The three-pronged approach I outlined might take some time before results are apparent, but it offers the possibility of a real cure. My 10-Day Gutbliss Plan (see Chapter 23) will certainly get you started on the path to bacterial balance, but if you have severe dysbiosis, rehabilitating your gut flora may take months or even years. Your microbiome wasn't built in a day—it took an entire lifetime. Getting it back to a state of bliss is a gradual process, but with the right approach, tangible improvements can almost always be made.

7

Uninvited Guests?

A FEW YEARS AGO, A VERY NICE WOMAN NAMED LUCY CAME TO SEE ME about some symptoms she was having. From the beginning she was convinced she had a parasite, and her story is in many ways representative of the trials and tribulations of figuring out whether that may indeed be the case.

Lucy had seen a number of gastroenterologists before me, and reading between the lines of their notes in her medical records, I could see they thought she was a little bit intense. She *was* a little bit intense, and rightly so. I would have been, too, if my life had been turned upside down by symptoms that no one could explain and that weren't getting any better.

In addition to bloating, she was also having fatigue, upper abdominal pain, nausea, and what she described as "weird" stools.

The first gastroenterologist Lucy saw did an upper endoscopy, thinking it might be acid reflux. The exam was normal other than a little redness in the stomach, which doctors often call "gastritis," which suggests inflammation of the stomach. But gastritis usually responds to treatment, and after being treated with acid suppressive medication for four weeks, Lucy was no better.

When stool studies for ova (eggs) and parasites came back negative from the first lab, I asked Lucy to use Popsicle sticks to scrape her stool into jars and send it off to a specialty lab in Arizona with an excellent track record for diagnosing parasites. When that lab didn't find anything unusual, we went ahead with a colonoscopy, with multiple biopsies in every segment to check for microscopic evidence of inflammation. When those biopsies came back normal, it was time to extend our investigation to the small intestine.

It can be hard to reach all twenty feet of small intestine between the stomach and colon; it's too long to completely examine with a traditional endoscope, but there are some novel ways to get a good look at it. A video capsule endoscope is a tiny capsule that packs a lot of punch—a camera, light source, radio transmitter, semiconductor, and an eight-hour battery—all in a pill the size of a large vitamin that's swallowed and flushable when it's excreted out the other end. One of my favorite tasks at work is reviewing the images obtained from the capsule as it travels through the intestines taking two pictures per second of everything in its field of view and condensing it into an incredible *Fantastic Voyage* video.

Lucy's video showed image after image of unremarkable small intestine. We had now examined her entire digestive tract, from her mouth to her anus, and it all looked normal. I decided to cast a broader net to explore whether the problem could be inside her abdomen but outside her intestines. But a CAT (computerized axial tomography) scan and MRI (magnetic resonance imaging) showed normal abdominal organs. Then I thought maybe the organs might look normal but not be working properly, so I ordered a scan to see how her gallbladder was functioning. When that came back normal, I ordered a gastric emptying study: a test where they give a person radio-labeled food to eat and then scan over the stomach to see how long it takes to empty. If a significant percentage of the meal is still in the stomach at the completion of the test, that's considered diagnostic for delayed emptying, a condition called gastroparesis, as mentioned in Chapter 3, that can cause bloating, pain, and nausea. That was normal, too.

Although neither of us wanted something to be wrong, we both knew something was, and we were desperate to find it. In the meantime, I asked Lucy to jump through a number of dietary hoops to see if any of them led to an improvement in her symptoms: gluten-free, dairy-free, no refined sugar, fructose-free, low-fat, no fat. She dutifully tried them all, to no avail.

During a visit to discuss all the tests we'd done, Lucy pulled out some photographs of her stool. There seemed to be an oily sheen to them, and she mentioned that some of them floated. While she didn't have any compelling reason for her pancreas to not be working properly, her stool and her symptoms fit the bill: oily-looking, foul-smelling stools that floated, crampy abdominal pain, bloating, and low-grade nausea—all symptoms consistent with a diagnosis of pancreatic insufficiency. I gave her a prescription for pancreatic replacement enzymes, feeling sure we had finally cracked the case.

No dice.

At a loss for what to do next, I asked Lucy to send one final set of stool specimens to the lab of a local infectious disease specialist who had a lot of expertise in parasitology. Lo and behold, they were positive for *Cyclospora*, a tiny one-celled organism transmitted by ingesting contaminated food or water, and best known for the 1996 outbreak associated with stool-tainted raspberries from Guatemala. *Cyclospora* usually causes diarrhea that can persist for several weeks. Additional symptoms include bloating, low-grade fever, abdominal cramping, poor appetite, weight loss, increased flatulence, vomiting, and fat malabsorption that results in oily, floating stools. Relapses are common if untreated.

Lucy finally got diagnosed not because of my amazing diagnostic skills (it certainly took me long enough), but because we both believed that something was wrong and were willing to roll up our sleeves and find it. Although she was treated and eventually got better, some people aren't so lucky. Parasites can live in the body undetected for years and, in addition to causing bloating, can create problems such as diarrhea, rectal itching, blood or mucus in the stool, low-grade fever, body aches, anemia, fat malabsorption, joint pain, teeth grinding, gallbladder dysfunction, and even neurological symptoms. Sometimes these symptoms don't resolve right away after treatment and they may require several rounds of therapy, particularly if your nutritional status is not ideal. The parasites themselves can also steal the nutrients in your food, consuming them before they get transported to your cells, leading to chronic malnutrition. Parasites have also been implicated in some other poorly understood conditions, many of which occur in tandem with irritable bowel syndrome (IBS), such as fibromyalgia and chronic fatigue syndrome.

Parasites are a lot more common than most people realize, affecting a huge number of people worldwide and up to a third of the population in the United States. Although many species are harmless and don't cause any symptoms, others can be a major cause of bloating. In this chapter I'll give you a sense of what to look for if you think a parasite might be responsible for your bloating, and what you can do about it.

Parasites Among Us

In my office I used to send stool specimens to a large commercial lab. Positive results for bacterial infections like *Salmonella* and *Campylobacter* were fairly common, but it was rare for the lab to ever identify a parasite. We had plenty of patients who worked overseas with the State Department, the Peace Corps, and international organizations, or who lived abroad and were visiting Washington. Was it possible that despite all the travel to sub-Saharan Africa and Southeast Asia, and all the complaints of bloating, diarrhea, fatigue, abdominal discomfort, and strange stools, so few people had been infected with a parasite? Or were we just looking in all the wrong places?

When we switched to a specialty lab—run by an infectious disease specialist—that focused exclusively on parasites (the same one that ultimately diagnosed Lucy), we suddenly started to get positive results. It was a valuable lesson and my first piece of advice for you: if you think you have a parasite, make sure your specimens (usually stool) are being sent to a reputable lab that has a good track record for parasite diagnosis. If the first test doesn't show anything and you're still convinced, get a second opinion somewhere else.

Conventional medicine would have you think parasites are rare, and mostly present in travelers or residents of exotic lands. Alternative medicine would have you think they're common and that, in fact, we're all infected. The truth is somewhere in the middle. The number of people infected with parasites worldwide varies dramatically, but reliable sources such the Centers for Disease Control and Prevention claim that the number is about 60 percent. Three types of parasites can infect the human digestive tract: tapeworms, roundworms (also known as nematodes), and protozoa. They range in size from microscopic to several feet long and can stay in the intestines or invade other distant organs. Some of these parasites are harmless species that don't lead to any problems, whereas others can cause acute and chronic symptoms. You may have wondered whether your bloating could be caused by a parasite, even if you've never visited the developing world. Here are two of the most common critters that can take up residence inside you.

CRYPTOSPORIDIUM

In 1993 there was an outbreak in the water supply in Milwaukee that infected over four hundred thousand people with a tiny one-celled microscopic organism called *Cryptosporidium* (*Crypto* for short). *Crypto* affects the small intestine, and the symptoms include bloating, cramps, diarrhea, fever, and dehydration. Although it's still unclear how the water supply got contaminated, runoff from cattle pastures was a likely explanation. *Cryptosporidium* oocysts that transmit infection are small enough to pass through some water filtration systems, including the Howard Avenue Water Purification Plant in Milwaukee. Oocysts are also hardy and resistant to chlorine and many other disinfectants, so they can survive in municipal water facilities. The fatalities in the Milwaukee outbreak were mostly people who were elderly or immune-compromised; AIDS patients were particularly at risk and constituted most of the one hundred deaths. As with many parasites, *Crypto* is spread through feces—either person to person, by inadvertent ingestion, or through contaminated objects like diapers, making day care centers and nursing homes breeding grounds for spreading infection.

GIARDIA

One-third of people living in less developed countries and between 2 and 8 percent in the more developed world have had giardiasis, one of the most common intestinal parasites affecting humans in the United States. Swallowing giardia cysts in contaminated food or water is the main method of acquiring the infection. Infectious cysts are then expelled in

Most Common Intestinal Parasites in the United States

- *Enterobius vermicularis* (pinworm)
- *Giardia lamblia* (giardia)
- *Ancylostoma duodenale* (Old World hookworm)
- *Necator americanus* (New World hookworm)
- *Entamoeba histolytica* (amebiasis)

Most Common Foodborne Parasites in the United States

- *Cryptosporidium*
- *Giardia intestinalis*
- *Cyclospora cayetanensis*
- *Toxoplasma gondii*
- *Entamoeba histolytica*

Most Common Intestinal Parasites Worldwide

- *Ascaris lumbricoides* (roundworm)
- Hookworm
- *Trichuris trichiuria* (whipworm)
- *Giardia intestinalis*
- *Strongyloides stercoralis* (threadworm)

feces, up to ten billion a day, although you only need a mere ten or so cysts to cause infection. Transmission is person to person or animal to person, with some cases being transmitted from dogs and other pets. Oral-anal sexual contact can result in high transmission rates. Symptoms usually appear a couple of weeks after exposure, and watery diarrhea or soft greasy stools are typical.

Gutbliss Solutions for Parasites

If you're exposed to a parasite, the likelihood of whether it will set up shop in your digestive tract and cause symptoms is, like other types of infections, related in part to how healthy your immune system is.

- A nourishing diet, lots of rest and exercise, and avoiding chemicals and other toxins are part of creating a healthy immune system and preventing parasites from taking hold.
- As is the case for bacteria, parasites have a sweet tooth, so limiting starchy, sugary foods can be an important part of preventing or treating a parasitic infection.
- Maintaining healthy levels of good bacteria in your gut by avoiding unnecessary antibiotics and drugs that change the pH will also help to discourage growth of parasites.
- Eating a high-fiber diet and taking a daily tablespoon of ground psyllium husk powder cleans out the intestines and can help to remove parasite eggs that may be attempting to make a home.
- Eating foods rich in vitamin A precursors, such as carrots and sweet potatoes, can help prevent parasitic larvae from penetrating, and raw garlic also has antiparasitic qualities.

Getting Rid of the Guests—and Their Baggage

The good news is that many parasitic infections are asymptomatic (i.e., there are no symptoms) or the symptoms are short-lived and resolve on their own without any treatment. The bad news is that parasites like giardia and many others can leave you with long-term symptoms, because they can be difficult to eradicate and some of the symptoms may continue even after the parasites are dead and out of your body. Bloating, low-grade nausea, burping, and fatigue can become chronic. Many of the patients I see in my office with chronic bloating recall having "Montezuma's Revenge" on spring break in Mexico or dysentery while on safari in

- Parasites can be transmitted from dogs and other pets, so make sure yours are regularly checked for worms and that their feces are properly disposed of. You also need to be on the lookout for whether your pet might be eating the infected stool of other animals, a practice that's not uncommon among puppies.
- To avoid coming into contact with infected stool, don't walk barefoot where animals have been.
- Wear gloves when gardening and make sure you're not watering vegetables with a contaminated water supply from a septic tank.
- Strict hand washing, careful washing of fruits and vegetables, filtering your drinking water, and avoiding raw and undercooked meat are also important preventive tactics. I've seen parasites in people doing a juice cleanse who weren't washing the produce well before juicing it.
- As much as I love them, salad bars can also be opportunities for contamination of food. One University of California study secretly observed a salad bar and found that over half the diners were in serious violation of the rules, using their fingers to sample the food and committing other hygiene transgressions.
- Poor sanitation in public or community spaces, especially in places such as nursing homes and day care centers, contributes to the spread of parasites.

southern Africa and now, months later, although the worst of their symptoms are over, they still don't feel quite right.

Some patients with parasites are misdiagnosed as suffering from IBS, without anyone ever considering that a parasite may be at the heart of their symptoms. (Note: That's different from being told you have postinfectious IBS, where the contribution of a previous infection is recognized.)

Figuring out which parasites are actually causing the symptoms and how to treat them is another gray area. In the medical literature, for example, *Blastocystis hominis* is often described as a harmless pathogen that doesn't need to be treated, but alternative medicine practitioners frequently recommend therapy. In my experience, a positive stool test for *Blastocystis hominis* is usually a sign that my patient has been exposed to other parasites as well, and treating the *Blastocystis hominis* if they have symptoms almost always leads to improvement.

If you think you have a parasite, it's always better to get diagnosed and figure out if you really do, and, if so, which specific one. The treatments can differ dramatically, from single-dose over-the-counter cures to weeks of prescription medication. There are lots of natural remedies, too, including things that may already be in your kitchen, like garlic, black walnuts, papaya seeds, and cloves. Wormwood tea is effective against many parasites and can be brewed at home, but it's not without potential side effects, including sleep disturbances and possible organ damage.

In the absence of a diagnosis, beware of signing up for Internet cures that may or may not work and could have unpleasant side effects you hadn't bargained on. You may ultimately need to see an infectious disease specialist or someone with expertise in parasitology. Be sure to ask when you make the appointment if they're familiar with diagnosing and treating parasites.

Parasites are common and although they're endemic in certain parts of the world, you don't need to travel to the developing world to pick one up. We all don't have parasites as the cause of our bloating, but some of us might. If you think you do, it's a good idea to investigate it. They're more common than many people realize and can cause a lot of different symptoms. A healthy immune system, which starts with a nourishing and balanced diet, is still one of your best defenses for preventing and eliminating these uninvited guests.

8

What's Happening
with Your Hormones?

IN MY PRACTICE, I SEE COUNTLESS WOMEN WHOSE METABOLISM SEEMS to have changed mysteriously and suddenly. Within a short period of time, they become chronically bloated, constipated, and fatigued, and they can't seem to stop gaining weight. If you're middle-aged and this sounds like you, you may be entering perimenopause, the period of time before menopause when, despite declining ovarian function, levels of the sex hormone estrogen that's made in the ovaries can actually start to climb in the female body. Perimenopause is characterized by irregular menstrual periods and usually lasts three to four years, but it can continue for up to a decade in some women. It's just one example of how hormones can interfere with your digestion, leading to bloating and discomfort. In this chapter you'll learn why hormones are so tightly linked to gut health, how they can affect you, and what you can do to lessen their impact.

Marvelous Messengers

Hormones are messengers that are made in your glands. They're released into your bloodstream and travel to millions of cells in your body, telling them what to do. The thyroid gland makes thyroid hormones that control your metabolism and a hormone called calcitonin that regulates calcium levels. Your ovaries are glands, too; they produce the sex hormones estrogen and progesterone and small amounts of testosterone and other male hormones. When everything works well, your hormones keep your body running smoothly, but out-of-control hormones can wreak havoc on your digestive system, not to mention the rest of your body.

THYROID HORMONES: MASTER MESSENGERS

Sherry had been diagnosed with an underactive thyroid—hypothyroidism—in her thirties, shortly after her second child was born, and had been on thyroid replacement therapy ever since. Her labs were checked by her endocrinologist every six months and, after she'd been on medication, they showed normal amounts of T3 and T4, the two main thyroid hormones. Her thyroid stimulating hormone (TSH), which is produced by the pituitary gland in the brain and tells the thyroid how much hormone to make, was also in the normal range. As a result of treatment, Sherry was what we call euthyroid, meaning she had adequate levels of thyroid hormones in her blood, even though in her case they were being supplied by a pill rather than by her thyroid gland.

If you have an underactive thyroid gland, your TSH will be high because your pituitary will be making and sending lots of TSH to your thyroid in an effort to stimulate it and get it to produce more T3 and T4.

If you have an overactive thyroid gland, your TSH will be low because your pituitary will sense the high circulating levels of T3 and T4 and turn down production of TSH.

If you have a normally functioning thyroid gland, your body continually assesses how much thyroid hormone is present and turns TSH production up or down accordingly. These are called feedback loops and are in place to prevent over- or underproduction, and to make sure that your body has access to the right amount of hormones depending on its needs.

While Sherry's labs consistently showed normal amounts of thyroid hormone, she didn't feel normal, and she hadn't in the last ten years since she was first diagnosed. Her initial symptoms had been bloating, exhaustion, constipation, low libido, feeling cold all the time, and weight gain. Her skin was dry and itchy, and she noticed she was losing the outer edges of her eyebrows. At first she thought her symptoms might be related to having just had a baby, but a year later, when things still hadn't improved and her bloating was worse, her doctor ordered blood work that revealed a poorly functioning thyroid gland.

The timing of her diagnosis wasn't that surprising. During pregnancy your body requires more thyroid hormone, so mild hypothyroidism that may not have been noticed before may become clinically apparent. Iodine deficiency is the most common cause of hypothyroidism worldwide, but autoimmune conditions like Hashimoto's thyroiditis are common around pregnancy, and hypothyroidism is much more common in women than men.

Sherry was started on the standard treatment: a synthetic form of T4 hormone replacement (levothyroxine), and she had been taking it ever since. While some of her symptoms had improved, she still felt puffy, bloated, and tired.

If your body were an airport, your thyroid gland would be air traffic control, secreting tiny bursts of hormone here and there to rev up your metabolism when you're busy and your body needs a boost, and dampening down production when you're asleep or at rest and need a little less. A pill once a day doesn't come close to replicating the body's natural ability to ramp up or down thyroid hormone production. Even when Sherry's dose was increased, she still felt lethargic and bloated.

An underactive thyroid gland slows down a lot of your bodily functions, including lymphatic drainage, leading to fluid retention and excess water weight. This causes a puffy feeling all over, particularly in your abdominal area, which is why bloating is so common. Hypothyroidism can also contribute to bloating by slowing down transit through the colon, causing constipation. Even when people are on thyroid replacement therapy, as Sherry was, the bloating and puffiness often remain.

Sherry wanted to know what else she could do to optimize her thyroid function and improve her bloating and constipation, since the medication didn't seem to be helping much with those symptoms. My experience with hypothyroidism and bloating is that medication rarely completely reverses the symptoms, even though it can improve them significantly. The hugely synergistic effect of diet *and* lifestyle, however, can't be emphasized enough. I recommended a gluten-free diet and cutting out other pro-inflammatory foods like refined sugar, as well as getting more regular exercise. My other recommendation was that she see a therapist for counseling and consider starting a meditation practice, since she was under a lot of stress—one of the exacerbating factors for thyroid disease.

WHEN THYROID PROBLEMS CAN BE ESPECIALLY HARD TO DETECT

If you're bloated and think a poorly functioning thyroid gland may be to blame, it's important to know that not all cases of thyroid dysfunction can be accurately diagnosed by a blood test. Your thyroid hormone levels may be within the normal range for the lab, but not for your body. There's also a condition called subclinical hypothyroidism, where the TSH is high, suggesting an underactive gland, but the levels of T4 and T3 are normal. This generally represents an early stage of hypothyroidism, but it's unclear whether treatment is always necessary. Since there's also a lot of debate about what constitutes a normal result with the existing tests, it may be helpful to see a specialist with experience in treating borderline thyroid dysfunction rather than initiating self-treatment with over-the-counter remedies, which, like prescription thyroid replacement therapy, can lead to heart palpitations, diarrhea, and anxiety if taken unnecessarily.

A PROBLEM ON THE RISE

For women over thirty, the risk of developing a thyroid disorder is almost 25 percent. The high sensitivity of the tests currently used is one explanation for that impressive number, but thyroid disease is definitely on the rise, and three main factors are likely to blame. The first is stress, which is very much a risk factor for immune-mediated forms of thyroid disease. The second is toxins in our environment: chemicals that act as endocrine disruptors and throw our glands and our bodies out of whack. The third is nutritional deficiencies based on our suboptimal diets, as well as iodine deficiency, low levels of selenium in the soil, fluorinated water, and eating too many processed soy products, which can cause an enlarged thyroid and slow function. These risk factors should be your guide as you think about how to prevent thyroid dysfunction or reverse existing disease.

Sex Hormones

Despite all the advances in women's rights, there's still a distinct tendency in health care to attribute symptoms in women to stress or anxiety. The very word *hysteria* is derived from the Greek word *hystera*, which means "uterus." We know that women suffer from real diseases, just as men do, and this bias toward ascribing their symptoms to emotions or stress often prevents real problems from being detected early and appropriately treated. That said, it's also true that there can be a hormonal component to symptoms like mood swings, altered libido, and bloating in women.

The menstrual cycle is divided into three phases: a follicular phase, followed by ovulation, and then the luteal phase. The follicular phase is defined by increasing amounts of estrogen, which stimulates the lining of the uterus to thicken and follicles, or immature eggs, to "ripen" in the ovaries. During ovulation, the dominant follicle in the ovary releases an ovum or egg, which lives for about a day if it isn't fertilized. In the luteal phase, the remains of the dominant follicle in the ovary, called a corpus luteum, produce large amounts of progesterone, which prime the uterus lining for implantation of a fertilized egg. In the absence of fertilization and implantation, both estrogen and progesterone levels drop, resulting in the uterus shedding its lining—the process of menstruation.

The different phases are associated with lots of other changes in your body in addition to what's happening in your uterus: body temperature fluctuations, altered libido, mood swings, changes in thyroid hormone production, neurological symptoms like migraines, and, of course, bloating. Fluctuating hormone levels lead to three changes that all cause bloating: an increase in intestinal gas production, an increase in water and salt retention by the kidneys, and a decrease in bile production. Bile helps to emulsify or break down fats and lubricate the small intestine. Low levels lead to accumulation of the products of digestion within the small intestine, causing bloating and constipation.

Estrogen is especially associated with water retention, which is why so many women experience bloating in the days leading up to their period as estrogen levels rise. Although progesterone has a diuretic effect, which can help with bloating, it also causes smooth muscle in your body, including your digestive tract, to relax, slowing down digestion and often leading to bloating, burping, and flatulence.

Menopause is associated with fluctuating estrogen levels and falling progesterone levels, which can both contribute to chronic bloating. There are a couple of important points to keep in mind regarding menopause. The first is that it occurs over a period of several years for some women, with gradual changes in hormone levels—what we refer to as perimenopause. So you might still be menstruating fairly regularly but having bloating and mood swings and not realize that it's due to the onset of menopause. The second is that the hormonal changes that accompany menopause aren't just limited to your reproductive organs; your entire body is different, including your metabolism and digestive system. Before menarche, which marks the beginning of menstruation, you can eat and tolerate most foods without gaining weight or experiencing gas. After menopause it can seem as if just looking at food makes you gain weight, and foods that were previously well tolerated may now cause gas and discomfort.

High levels of estrogen also affect where the body distributes fat, causing more deposition of fat in the abdominal area. If you're not sure whether your expanding waistline is due to bloat or belly fat, measuring your waist throughout your menstrual cycle can help. If it's bloat, your waist measurement will vary by more than an inch; if it's belly fat, there'll be little variation.

Eating smaller meals with fewer calories, reducing salt intake, and engaging in regular strenuous exercise are key to preventing weight gain and bloating in the perimenopausal period. (These strategies are helpful if you experience significant premenstrual syndrome [PMS] symptoms, too.)

I see so many women in this age group who don't understand why they're bloated and gaining weight, since they've made no changes in their diet and exercise routines. That's actually why they're having problems—because they haven't made the compensatory changes needed to accommodate their changing hormonal milieu.

THE CHALLENGES OF ESTROGEN DOMINANCE

As you approach menopause, levels of both progesterone and estrogen may decline, but progesterone decreases more than estrogen, leading to a state of estrogen dominance, a condition highly correlated with bloating. Three additional factors can contribute to estrogen dominance in women.

1. Exposure to xenoestrogens—compounds produced outside the body that have an estrogenic effect. Xenoestrogens are endocrine disruptors. They create hormonal imbalance in your endocrine and reproductive organs, and they're widespread in the environment: in hormones given to some commercially raised animals, in pesticides used on produce, and in lots of the plastics and chemicals in everyday use. The universality of xenoestrogens in industrialized countries may be one of the reasons we're seeing earlier onset of menarche (i.e., onset of periods) and so much breast and reproductive cancer.
2. Obesity contributes to estrogen dominance because a hormone called androstenedione, made in the ovaries and adrenal glands, gets converted to estrogen by fat cells.
3. Stress, which depletes progesterone levels, worsens estrogen dominance.

Birth control pills (BCP) and hormone replacement therapy (HRT) are also forms of xenoestrogens and a major cause of bloating. Weight loss on a high-estrogen BCP may be extremely challenging due to fluid and salt retention as well as weight gain. Many doctors believe these pills cause some degree of insulin resistance, a condition that can interfere with your ability to lose weight, especially if you eat a lot of carbohydrates. If you already have a tendency toward insulin resistance or are prediabetic, you may be more likely to gain weight from BCP. Using an alternative form of birth control or choosing a BCP with the lowest amount of estrogen possible makes sense if you're worried about bloating or weight gain. Low-dose BCP containing 20 micrograms of estrogen are among the lowest on the market. Weight gain of more than 5 percent of total body weight after starting BCP may be a sign of insulin resistance and should prompt a discussion with your doctor about a glucose tolerance test to diagnose it. Ironically, going off BCP can lead to bloating and constipation due to ovulation starting again, especially if you've been on the pill for a long time.

If you're menopausal and bloated, HRT may seem like the solution. Although HRT can help alleviate other menopause-related symptoms, its

Gutbliss Solutions for Estrogen Dominance

PMS, menstrual disturbances, ovarian cysts, endometriosis (tissue from the uterus present outside the uterine cavity), and fibroids (noncancerous tumors of the uterus that originate from the smooth muscle layer) are all associated with estrogen dominance and they all cause bloating—so treating estrogen dominance is key in getting bloating under control if you have one of these conditions. How do you treat estrogen dominance?

- Eat organic produce that hasn't been treated with synthetic pesticides or chemicals.
- Avoid eating commercially raised animals that have been given hormones.
- Don't use plastic water bottles.
- Use gloves when you come into contact with household cleaners and solvents.
- Consider forms of birth control other than hormonal methods like the pill.
- Think about forgoing hormone replacement therapy.

estrogenic effect usually makes bloating worse—and there are other associated potential health risks, such as cancer, heart disease, stroke, and blood clots.

A number of other conditions that involve the uterus and ovaries can be associated with bloating and hormonal imbalance. Many of the women I see with bloating have polycystic ovary syndrome (PCOS), which is associated with high levels of androgens and affects 5 to 10 percent of women of reproductive age. Classic symptoms include excessive facial hair, male-pattern baldness, acne, obesity, irregular menses, decreased fertility, and insulin resistance. Most but not all women with PCOS will have multiple ovarian cysts demonstrated on ultrasound. Some studies have raised the possibility that obesity causes PCOS rather than the other way around. What we do know is that addressing insulin resistance and obesity through a diet that restricts gluten and refined sugar improves a lot of the symptoms of PCOS, including bloating. In fact, I've seen high androgen (male hormone) levels, infertility, and irregular menstrual patterns in PCOS resolve with dietary modification and weight loss.

The digestive and reproductive systems are next-door neighbors, so it's not surprising that times of hormonal change like menstruation and menopause can be associated with significant bloating. Recognizing that your body may have different requirements during these life phases is an important part of getting the symptoms under control. Estrogen dominance is hard to avoid if you live in the industrialized world, but there are choices you can make that will help to restore your hormonal balance, alleviate your bloating, and improve your reproductive health.

9

Was It Good for You?
Sex and the Bloat

WE'RE TOLD THAT A DECREASE IN LIBIDO IS A NATURAL PART OF AGING, but in my practice a lot of the women who are having bedroom issues are in their twenties and thirties. If you're bloated and also not in the mood, there may be a connection between the two. Anatomically, the bowels and pelvic organs are next-door neighbors, and both depend on a well-balanced ecosystem to function properly. Bacterial imbalance, constipation, and bloating can upset both your digestive and your gynecological health.

It's a good idea to share what's going on with your doctor and have a thorough physical exam. Excluding systemic diseases like diabetes, Crohn's, or hypothyroidism, which can affect multiple systems, is an important part of exploring the connection between gut problems and lack of libido. Stress can also play a significant role in both digestive and sexual dysfunction, so taking a closer look at your mental health may also be helpful. In this chapter I'll shed some light on the connection between your sex life and your bloating and give you some practical advice on how to improve both.

Jane has been married for two years. She's in her midtwenties, gorgeous, and the picture of health. She works in sales and spends much of her day with clients. Daily meetings require form-fitting dresses or suits, and her petite size 2 frame is unforgiving. Her bloat has nowhere to hide. She told me about a weekend wedding she and her husband had recently attended: "I woke up with a flat abdomen and feeling fine, but by evening disaster had struck—I looked six months pregnant and couldn't come close to fitting into the dress I'd brought to wear to the wedding!"

Now, lots of people say they look six months pregnant and then lift up their clothes to reveal a mostly flat belly with maybe just a hint of a paunch. But Jane had brought photos of the wedding—and she really did look like she was just a few months away from delivering.

Thinking her problem might be lactose intolerance, Jane had tried avoiding dairy for a few weeks, but it didn't make any difference. When she first came to see me, she was four months into a vegan experiment, but still bloated and despondent. She was also constipated, barely able to push out a hard stool two or three times a week.

In addition to not looking and feeling her best, only two years into her marriage her sex life was already beginning to suffer. Her protruding abdomen wasn't a deterrent for her husband; the issue was, as she put it: "I'm just stuffed!" Everything from the waist down felt full to capacity, and she couldn't bear the thought of anything else going in. She also confided that she was deathly afraid of passing gas during sex, which had happened a few times, and her pelvic muscles were now clenched so tight that penetration had become awkward and painful. Tearfully she recounted her avoidance tactics for deferring sex, her husband's growing frustration, and the toll it was taking on their marriage.

The cause of Jane's bloating was relatively easy to figure out once I took a detailed history. She'd been on antibiotics for Lyme disease as a teenager for a full year. Over time, the antibiotics had killed off not only the "bad bacteria" responsible for her Lyme disease, but also lots of the "good bacteria" in her digestive tract, causing dysbiosis, or bacterial imbalance. An overabundance of undesirable species was producing large amounts of methane and hydrogen gas, causing terrible bloating.

Being bloated and gassy made it difficult for Jane to get aroused, so her vagina was dry and hard to penetrate. But there was another reason she was having so much burning and discomfort with sex. Jane's bacterial overgrowth wasn't just in her gut; it was in her vagina, too. Over the years, as her GI tract had become overpopulated with unfriendly bacteria, so had her vaginal flora. The burning she was now experiencing with intercourse was a direct result of that bacterial imbalance. Her gynecologist had checked for sexually transmitted diseases and done several cultures. Each time the results came back showing "heavy bacterial growth" and she was given a diagnosis of BV—bacterial vaginosis. She didn't have any vaginal discharge but she did have a characteristic fishy odor, especially after sex, which added to her embarrassment and made oral sex completely off-limits. She had taken three rounds of antibiotics, which were supposed to treat BV, but nothing had changed.

Antibiotics may temporarily improve things if you have BV or dysbiosis of the gut, but for most people it's a shortsighted fix because antibiotics can actually contribute to the problem and make things worse in the long term. There are no antibiotics that selectively kill off only harmful bacteria. In fact, even the antibiotics prescribed to treat bacterial overgrowth often end up contributing to it by killing off large amounts of essential good bacteria, too.

In addition to conflict in her microbiome, Jane had another complication from her bloating that was making her sex life suffer. Anatomically, the rectum sits just behind the vagina, and the two are separated by less than half a centimeter. Jane's constipation and straining had led to a condition called a rectocele, where the wall of her rectum was bulging and pressing against her vagina and filling with stool, leaving less room for her husband's penis and causing dyspareunia—painful intercourse.

Jane ate a balanced diet, but she still wasn't getting enough fiber or drinking enough water. I started her on a twice-daily heaping tablespoon of ground psyllium husk powder dissolved in a large glass of water and made her buy a one-liter glass bottle to start measuring her water consumption. Within a week she was having more frequent and softer bowel movements, but sex was still as painful as ever. Jane had been living with painful intercourse for so long that her brain and body had begun to expect pain during sex. Anticipation of the discomfort was making it difficult for her to relax her pelvic muscles, which of course made things even more painful.

Pelvic floor biofeedback using special sensors in the vagina, in addition to internal pelvic muscle massage, helped tremendously with getting

Gutbliss Solutions for Dysbiosis and Bacterial Vaginosis (BV)

The most effective way to treat dysbiosis is a three-pronged approach: avoidance, encouragement, and repopulation.

1. *Avoid* antibiotics and other drugs that contribute to the problem, including antacids, acid suppressors, and steroids.
2. *Encourage* the growth of good bacteria by consuming prebiotics—high-fiber foods that literally feed your good bugs, including foods such as kale, spinach, oats, artichokes, asparagus, garlic, and leeks. Fermented foods such as sauerkraut and cabbage also increase the numbers of good bacteria. Staying away from sugary, starchy foods that favor proliferation of bad bacteria, which thrives on "eating" sugar, is a must.
3. *Repopulate* your gut or vagina with large amounts of live bacteria in the form of a robust probiotic. Probiotics are taken orally in the form of a pill, powder, or liquid.

It may take several months before you see meaningful results, but this approach offers the possibility of a real cure for dysbiosis and BV, rather than an antibiotic Band-Aid that ultimately ends up being part of the problem.

Jane's pelvic muscles to relax. The practitioner to whom I referred Jane was extraordinarily kind and compassionate and makes all of her patients feel at ease, which is essential when you're teaching them how to massage their vaginal and rectal muscles. She also taught Jane how to do guided meditation using deep breathing techniques before intercourse to help her relax.

Although Jane's constipation had improved and her pelvic muscles were much more relaxed, her rectocele was still a problem. It was regularly filling with stool and sometimes required her to insert a finger vaginally and press on it through the wall of the vagina to get the contents to empty. A radiology test called defecography (in which the rectum is filled with material containing a contrast dye) showed an extremely large bulge that filled up and didn't empty as the rest of the material was expelled.

X-ray images clearly showed how Jane's bulging rectum was pressing on her vagina.

I referred Jane to a colorectal surgeon who agreed she would benefit from surgical repair of the rectocele. The surgery involved reinforcing the connective fibrous tissue between the vagina and the rectum to support the rectum and push it up and away from the vagina. Things healed nicely and follow-up testing showed resolution of the rectocele. And since Jane's dietary and bowel habits were better and her pelvic muscles more relaxed, I was optimistic about the rectocele not recurring.

Ultimately, the combination of rebalancing Jane's gut and vaginal flora, improving her constipation, repairing her rectocele, and helping her and her pelvic muscles to relax led to tremendous improvements in the bedroom. Sex was no longer something uncomfortable that she dreaded, and as her bloating improved, she was less self-conscious and didn't require the room to be completely dark or her belly to be covered. It had taken a while to sort things out, but the results were definitely worth it!

If you're bloated and feel like it's affecting your sex life, I encourage you to look for explanations and solutions. I hope you find the answer to what's bloating you somewhere within the pages of this book, and if things get better in the bedroom as a result, I'll be doubly delighted.

Gutbliss Solutions to Get You in the Mood

If you've wondered whether your bloating could be interfering with your sex life, here are some factors to consider with your gynecologist and some suggestions that might improve things:

- Investigate the possibility that mechanical issues like a rectocele, scar tissue, or uterine fibroids may be contributing to your bloating and making sex painful.
- Ask about pelvic floor disorders, especially if you have trouble pushing out stool and difficulty relaxing your pelvic muscles during intercourse. A good rectal and pelvic exam may help your doctor figure it out, but you may also need more investigation with an ultrasound where a probe is

inserted vaginally (transvaginal ultrasound) or tests that can check the pressure in the rectum (anorectal manometry) and show the relationship between the rectum and the vagina during bowel movements (defecography).

- If you are clenched tight down below and sex is painful, a good biofeedback practitioner with experience in pelvic floor disorders may help you relax your pelvic muscles, which should improve things a lot.

- Remember that bacterial imbalance in the gut can also mean bacterial imbalance in your vagina, which can cause discomfort with sex and decrease your libido. Rather than reaching for the quick fix of an antibiotic, consider a more long-term and effective approach to restoring balance that involves a change in diet and a probiotic.

- Having a rectum full of stool that's trying to come out can make you feel toxic and definitely affect your libido. A good bowel movement is the ultimate detox, and it can also be a potent aphrodisiac. If you're constipated:

  - Add some ground psyllium husk powder to create a bulkier stool that's easier to pass.
  - Increase the amount of fiber in your diet from fruits and vegetables.
  - Make sure you're getting enough water and exercise to help keep things moving.
  - A regular cleanse with green juices and psyllium husk may leave you feeling light and relaxed and do wonders for both your digestive health and your sex life. For more on how to do this, see my 10-Day Gutbliss Plan in Chapter 23.
  - Try to have a bowel movement and pass gas before sex. This might take some planning, but feeling light and well cleaned out usually makes sex more enjoyable.
  - Think about when the best time for sex is for your body—it may not be at night when your colon is filled with an entire day's worth of food and there's a liter of gas brewing above it. Consider having sex in the morning, when most people's bloating is at its best. Tricky, but not impossible, with kids. If early-morning action doesn't work for you, then try to eat light on the days when you plan to have sex, and

try not to have sex immediately after eating, especially at night. You'll be full and uncomfortable and more likely to pass gas. Stomach rumbling from delaying your meal won't spoil the mood as much as smelly gas.

- Think about different positions. Your partner spooning you from behind rather than on top of you may be more comfortable, especially if you have a full colon.

- If you think you may be depressed, anxious, or overly stressed, have your mental health assessed by a professional, especially if you've been diagnosed with irritable bowel syndrome and told that stress is partly to blame. Researchers frequently make reference to the "second brain" in the gut—the millions of nerve cells in the digestive tract that allow us to "feel" the inner world of our gut. The gut-brain interaction is essential for good digestive health, and I suspect a similar relationship exists between the pelvic organs and the brain. Not feeling well psychologically makes it much more challenging for you to have a healthy sex life.

10

Belly Fat or Bloated?

BLOATING CONSULTATIONS COME IN ALL SHAPES AND SIZES. I SEE SLENder people with protruding, bloated abdomens, and people who are overweight but have additional distention from bloating. Every now and again I'll see skinny patients with a big belly who are complaining about being bloated, and I have the awkward task of breaking the news that their out-of-proportion midsection isn't bloating—it's belly fat.

How can you tell? In this chapter you'll learn the differences between bloating and belly fat and my foolproof way to distinguish between the two, as well as what I'm checking for when I examine the abdomen. I'll explain the genetics and the dangers behind being an "apple" rather than a "pear" in terms of body shape and what, if anything, you can do about it.

Insulin is the hormone you definitely need to be familiar with if you're battling the belly bulge, especially if you're concerned about diabetes, heart disease, or cancer. I'll reveal my realistic strategies for keeping insulin levels low and explain why calorie counting is for the birds, especially when it comes to belly fat.

Okay, So What's the Difference?

First, the burning question: how can you tell bloating from belly fat? Bloating is usually caused by gas (and sometimes fluid), and it generally ebbs and flows—some mornings you're as flat as a board and then by dinnertime you look six months pregnant. Or things are fine for a while and then you have several days when you can't button your pants. Occasionally a solid mass in the uterus, ovaries, or colon presents as bloating and causes constant, if not increasing, protrusion of the abdomen, but that's the exception, not the norm. For most people, there is lots of variation in their bloating.

If you're not sure whether your bulge is bloat or belly fat, this may help you figure it out: measure around your waist using a tape measure first thing in the morning and at bedtime every day for several days in a row. If you're bloated, you'll typically see that the number varies quite a bit. If you have belly fat masquerading as bloat, the measurement shouldn't change by more than an inch.

While you have the measuring tape out, I want you to use it for another super-important number: your waist-to-height ratio, also known as the index of central obesity. I know it sounds very official and a little scary, but you absolutely need to know this number and here's why: if your waist circumference is more than half your height, even if you're not overweight, you may have more belly fat than you thought, and that could be a real problem.

What I Do When a Patient Comes to Me Complaining of Bloat

In my office I have massage tables instead of traditional examination tables. I'd rather people think relaxation than rectal exam when they come to see me, although the reality is that they often get both. Here's how I approach the exam and what I'm looking, listening, and feeling for.

LOOKING (INSPECTION)

With inspection I'm checking the overall appearance of the abdomen as well as looking for more specific things—lumps or bumps that might suggest an underlying mass, prominent surface veins or yellowing of the skin that could be a sign of liver disease, or areas of increased pigmentation from undiagnosed diabetes.

Sometimes the abdomen is flat from the belly button up but the lower part looks distended, suggesting a full colon. Constipated patients tend to store their stool in the sigmoid colon, which is in the lower left part of the abdomen. Sometimes I can see a bulge there, even before I confirm it with my hands.

Inspection is also when I first start to get a sense of whether I'm dealing with air, fluid, or fat. If you're lying down, air floats to the top of the abdomen while fluid tracks to the sides, causing bulging flanks. Fat tends to encircle the waist like a tube, without much positional movement, and unlike air, I can see it in the back when the patient sits up.

LISTENING (AUSCULTATION)

Auscultation is when I listen to the bowel sounds, which aren't usually affected by bloating unless someone has gastroparesis—delayed emptying of the stomach (see Chapter 3)—where sloshing of the contents can be heard when I place the stethoscope over the stomach and rock the patient gently from side to side. A complete or partial intestinal blockage can cause bloating and high-pitched or completely absent bowel sounds.

FEELING (PALPATION)

Palpation is when I touch and feel the abdomen, and this is when I gather more evidence for bloating or belly fat (or both). To palpate the abdomen, I move my hands in a clockwise direction, applying pressure as I go, feeling to make sure organs aren't enlarged, checking for masses that could represent an underlying cancer, and locating any pockets of fluid or gas. I'm also evaluating for tenderness that might suggest underlying inflammation. If I press deeply on the lower left side in constipated patients, I can usually find bowel filled with stool that feels like a fat sausage rolling around under my fingers.

SOUNDING (PERCUSSION)

It's during the last part of the exam, percussion, where I'm able to confirm bloating versus belly fat. When I put my left hand over the abdomen and tap lightly on it with the fingers of my right hand, it makes a sound. A dull sound indicates solid tissue or fluid, whereas air-filled bowels sound like a drum—a phenomenon we call tympany.

Apple or Pear, and Why It Matters

My patient Lisa is the prototypic apple shape: petite, with very thin arms and legs and a soft, wide midsection. If you lined up all the women in her family and covered their faces, you wouldn't be able to tell them apart—they all have the identical "apple" body type.

Those of us with generous hips, butts, and legs are correspondingly classified as "pears." Is whether we end up an apple or a pear simply the luck of the draw, or is there a genetic component, as Lisa's family tree would suggest?

The Genetic Investigation of Anthropometric Traits consortium is an international collaboration of over four hundred scientists that researches the various genes associated with body fat distribution and obesity. A few years ago the group identified thirteen new areas with variations in the DNA that correlated with whether people were apple- or pear-shaped. Although the identified genes only explained variations in fat distribution in about 1 percent of the population, the research suggests that for some of us, particularly women, specific biological mechanisms may play a role in determining where fat is stored in our body.

Besides your genes, risk factors for being an apple include toxins in the environment, increased consumption of fructose, estrogens in foods like soy products, chemicals that affect the endocrine system, and some prescription drugs like steroids.

Having love handles versus thunder thighs doesn't just determine what sorts of clothes look good on you; it can also predict your likelihood of developing certain diseases. The condition known as metabolic syndrome, present in up to 25 percent of the U.S. population, is a deadly combination of risk factors that dramatically increases your chances of developing heart disease, stroke, diabetes, and some types of cancer. Those risk factors include high blood pressure, high fasting blood sugar, increased waist circumference, low levels of HDL ("good" cholesterol), and elevated triglycerides. Triglycerides are the main constituents of animal fats and vegetable oils, and high levels have been linked to heart disease and stroke.

If you have an apple shape, you're much more likely to have metabolic syndrome, although it's not the superficial muffin-top belly fat under the skin that's the problem; it's the deeper visceral fat. If you take a peek inside an apple-shaped abdomen, you're likely to see butter-colored bundles of visceral fat wrapped around the abdominal organs.

Visceral fat isn't just a harmless glob of yellow stuff; it's a complex tissue similar in function to other endocrine organs, such as the thyroid gland. In addition to affecting the function of the liver, pancreas, and other internal organs, visceral fat itself is hormonally active, producing estrogens, proteins, and other substances that can affect insulin levels, blood sugar, cholesterol, and even the reproductive system. Belly fat puts you at higher risk for elevated lipids (fats) in the blood, diabetes, breast cancer, colon cancer, gallbladder problems, high blood pressure, and lots of other health issues, likely related to the hormonally active substances it secretes.

Lisa, my "apple" patient, developed gestational diabetes when she was pregnant, which never resolved. The risk of developing type 2 diabetes is seven times higher in women with gestational diabetes than those without, so this wasn't too surprising. What was surprising was that she was an avid runner, was a great cook, and ate a healthy diet. Her good habits were probably what had held diabetes at bay until a fifty-pound weight gain during her pregnancy and hormonal changes got the best of her. Thirteen years after the birth of her daughter, her blood sugar was still well controlled on just oral medication, and she had no complications of diabetes (such as kidney or eye problems).

Her biggest frustration was that no matter what she did, she just couldn't get rid of her belly. Tired of the solid spare tire around her waist that never went flat, Lisa was hell-bent on liposuction—a procedure I never recommend, especially in diabetics, for whom the procedure carries additional risks.

Not Loving Liposuction

During liposuction, small incisions are made in the skin and a thin, hollow tube is inserted to loosen the fat and suction it out. Here's why sucking or cutting out parts of your body that you don't like is not a good idea. There are a constant number of fat cells in your body. While it's rare to lose fat cells, there are a few times in life when you may actually gain them, including in utero before you're even born, and at puberty. When you gain weight, the cells don't usually multiply, but instead swell to several times their normal size. When you lose weight, the cells decrease in size, but the number of cells tends to remains constant. Researchers at Mount Sinai Hospital in New York City found that fat cells can die but they're usually replaced: the remaining fat seems to tell the body to make more fat cells to keep the number constant.

When you remove fat via liposuction, the same thing often happens. The fascinating thing is that the fat doesn't necessarily come back in the area from which it was removed. It can come back in totally different places! In a study by Robert Eckel, MD, at the University of Colorado, women who had liposuction of the lower abdomen, hips, or thighs were followed for a year. The results showed re-accumulation of fat in the upper abdomen and triceps, not the areas where the fat had originally been removed.

There was another striking result in Dr. Eckel's study. Up to five liters of fat, the maximal recommended amount, was removed from the liposuction group. Six weeks after the procedure, body fat in the liposuction group had decreased by 2.1 percent and by only 0.28 percent in a comparison group not receiving liposuction. But one year later, there was no difference in body fat between the two groups.

And finally: fat that came back in the different areas wasn't just the subcutaneous fat under the skin; it was also the deeper visceral fat associated with heart disease.

Eating Your Way Out of Belly Fat

Once I explained the data to Lisa about fat returning post-liposuction, she was less enthused about liposuction and more willing to consider a radical change in her diet—not just what she ate but when she ate it.

WHEN TO EAT

Because she was frequently on a diet, Lisa skipped meals a lot, especially early in the day when she was busy getting her daughter ready for school and at work when things started to pile up. Lisa's usual pattern was to skip breakfast and lunch, and then munch on cheese and crackers while she was preparing dinner.

My first piece of advice for Lisa was to eat at more consistent intervals. In general, I'm not a stickler about the three-meals-a-day principle. How much you eat should be based on your energy needs. Some people clearly have greater energy expenditures and needs than others.

Also, if you eat a big dinner most nights and then go right to bed, chances are you don't need to eat a big breakfast first thing in the morning. But if you skip breakfast, I have one important stipulation: you need to have nutritious food available when you get hungry later in the day. If not, your body is going to send you in search of quick energy, and that usually means sugar, not nutrients.

Having nourishing food available generally involves preparing it ahead of time and taking it with you. It makes sense that you need to eat when you most need the calories. So unless you work the night shift, that's during the day, not at eight p.m. when the busy part of your day is over and you're much less active. That's sort of like trying to drive your car around all day with an empty tank and then filling it up at night right before you park it in the garage. Not an efficient way to drive.

WHAT TO EAT

Next we had to address what kinds of foods Lisa was eating. Her teenage daughter had a passion for pasta, so that was frequently what they had for dinner, with French bread, a salad, or steamed vegetables. Other nights it was fish with rice and veggies or roast chicken and mashed potatoes.

Crackers and pretzels were in heavy rotation before and after dinner. Definitely not junk food, but for Lisa, not a regimen that was helping her get rid of belly fat. She needed help decoding the mystery of what she should be eating.

To add to the challenge, Lisa was perimenopausal—a time when changes in estrogen levels cause fat deposition to shift so that apples and pears alike may find themselves with a shrinking tush and an expanding midsection. You can't spot-reduce in specific areas like your belly, but if most of your extra fat is deposited around your middle, then that's where most of it will come from when you start to lose weight. Lisa had certainly experienced this firsthand—the only time her belly had gone down was when she had starved herself down twenty pounds from 135 to 115. This time, we were trying to get her belly down without starvation tactics. In order to do that, there was one very important factor we were going to have to consider.

Like many people with belly fat, Lisa was very insulin resistant. Any regimen we came up with was going to have to take that into account.

Insulin Resistance: The Crash Course

Insulin resistance is a condition in which certain cells in the body fail to respond to the effects of the hormone insulin. Insulin is the key that unlocks the doors to the cells and allows glucose to enter so the cells can use it as an energy source. With insulin resistance the key doesn't fit well, so the door doesn't open properly, some of the glucose can't enter the cells, and the level of unused glucose in the blood rises. The pancreas, the organ that makes insulin, produces more and more of it in an effort to get the rising blood glucose levels under control, but eventually the pancreas just can't keep up. Type 2 diabetes occurs when this compensatory increase in insulin secretion by the pancreas fails. (With type 1 diabetes, the insulin-producing cells of the pancreas are destroyed and can't produce any insulin at all, leading to very high levels of glucose in the blood that have to be treated by injecting insulin.)

Insulin resistance and type 2 diabetes can often be controlled by diet rather than with medication. The key is figuring out what to eat and, believe it or not, that actually has nothing to do with calories. Take the ex-

The Not-So-Sweet Skinny on Artificial Sweeteners

There are lots of good reasons to avoid artificial sweeteners. They're a common cause of bloating because they're not absorbed in the small intestine and undergo fermentation by colonic bacteria, which produces a lot of gas. Some of them have been linked to cancer, autoimmune diseases, neurological symptoms, and other problems. They can also increase insulin levels. That's because insulin is released in response to sweetness, not calories, and artificial sweeteners are plenty sweet. In fact, in some studies diet sodas are a bigger risk factor for obesity than regular soda, despite the zero calorie advertising. Researchers have consistently found that there's a correlation between drinking diet soda and being overweight. Now maybe that's because overweight people tend to drink more diet soda in an attempt to lose weight, but it also raises the possibility of a contribution to elevated insulin levels and the creation of more sugar cravings by these substances.

The San Antonio Heart Study analyzed the dietary habits of over five thousand people and found that people who drank sugar-sweetened soda and diet soda both gained weight, but the diet soda drinkers gained more, and the more diet sodas they consumed, the more weight they gained. The now-famous Framingham Heart Study, one of the longest-running, intergenerational studies of cardiovascular disease, found a link between both sugar-sweetened soda and diet soda and metabolic syndrome, suggesting that increased insulin levels were a side effect of both.

Another concern is that artificial sweeteners may condition people to want to eat more sweet foods. Sweetness is an addictive habit, regardless of whether that sweet flavor is from sugar or some other substance. Although I'm an advocate of carefully watching your sugar consumption, when it comes to sweeteners, I always recommend calories over chemicals.

ample of artificial sweeteners. Because she almost never ate dessert, Lisa thought she was being "good" about her diet. But she drank two diet sodas a day and used a packet of artificial sweetener in each of her three cups of coffee. One of the common mistakes people with insulin resistance make is using artificial sweeteners. As a physician, I'm in favor of technology, but no matter how advanced our science gets, some principles still hold true, and one fundamental is that you can't cheat Mother Nature. Sweetness without calories, and without any undesirable side effects? I don't believe it, and the research doesn't bear it out, either.

Lisa's caloric intake was on the low side, but she ate a lot of rice, potatoes, and crackers, and she complained of feeling hungry all the time. Decreasing her insulin requirement was part of the master plan, and to do that, we needed to decrease the foods (and drinks) that were increasing her glucose levels. I'm generally not a huge fan of low-carbohydrate diets; most people regain the weight quickly, and there's much more fluid loss than fat loss in the early stages. As motivating and exciting as it is to see the scale drop by eight pounds in a week, it can be just as disappointing to watch it go up by three pounds after one bowl of pasta. And while no calorie counting is required, there's no deviating from the list of allowed foods without weighty consequences. Even more important, although low-carbohydrate doesn't necessarily mean high-protein, these diets can encourage overconsumption of disease-causing high-fat animal protein.

That said, given Lisa's diabetic profile and her high-carb habits, lowering her intake of processed carbohydrates was critical to weight control, but it was important to find the right regimen. Low-carbohydrate diets can be successful in the short term but problematic long-term; in extremely low-carb diets, the body can enter ketosis, when it starts to burn fat for energy in the absence of the glucose it's missing from the diet, and this in turn can lead to kidney problems and lots of physical complaints. Avoiding these kinds of extremes, plus steering clear of the high animal fat option, means picking and choosing a very particular kind of low-carbohydrate approach.

Eat Like a Cavewoman?

The Paleo diet, sometimes called the caveman, Stone Age, or hunter-gatherer diet, recommends that we eat the way our ancestors in the Paleolithic era did, before agriculture and grains were introduced. Since none of us were around to actually observe what our Paleolithic ancestors were consuming, much in the Paleo dogma is speculative. The emphasis is on fish, poultry, meats, wild game, fruits, vegetables, root vegetables, nuts, and seeds, and excludes dairy, grains, refined sugar, legumes, and processed oils. As far as low-carb regimens go, the fact that unlimited amounts of fruits and vegetables are allowed on this plan is a plus. Low-carb diets often discourage fruits, and many people limiting carbohydrates will overcompensate with meat, which puts them at risk for other problems, such as heart disease and cancer.

It's still totally possible, if not likely, to overdo the animal protein consumption on a Paleo diet, and I suspect our Paleolithic ancestors ate far less meat than most modern-day Paleo devotees. It's also important to keep in mind that most people whose health improves on a low-carb regimen get better because they're eliminating processed carbohydrates and refined sugars, not because they're including meat.

Slow Carb Solution

After discussing various options, we decided on a modified version of a "slow carb" regimen for Lisa, which allowed healthy sources of carbohydrates like beans, quinoa, brown rice, sweet potatoes, and yams, but excluded refined sugars, high-fat dairy, gluten, and some other processed grains. There was still plenty to eat, and she didn't miss snacking on cheese and crackers since she could snack on raw unsalted nuts and hummus or guacamole with vegetables. Her meals were now mostly fish or chicken with an array of vegetables, plus a salad and half a sweet potato, or beans and vegetables over brown rice.

Getting with the Glycemic Index

In 1981 David Jenkins, MD, PhD, and research chair in the Department of Nutritional Sciences at the University of Toronto, wrote a paper on which foods were most ideal for people with diabetes, and the effect of carbohydrates on blood sugar. This study became the basis for the glycemic index (GI), a measure of how much each gram of carbohydrate in a specific food increases blood sugar. Glucose, to which all other foods were compared, was arbitrarily assigned a value of 100. Carbohydrates that are easily digested and rapidly broken down into simple sugars have a high GI, whereas

Gutbliss Solutions for Belly Fat

When it comes to reducing belly fat:

- The quality of what you're eating can be more important than the quantity.
- Eliminating carbohydrates altogether is much too extreme and not healthy. Instead, seek out nutritious carbs from sources like fruits, vegetables, legumes, nuts, seeds, yams, sweet potatoes, brown rice, and quinoa.
- Get rid of artificial sweeteners.
- Tone and strengthen your abdominal muscles through core exercises.
- Control stress. High cortisol levels caused by stress are a major contributor to belly fat.

All of these strategies will help to keep insulin levels in check, keep metabolic syndrome at bay, and decrease belly fat. It's hard to completely change your body type, but you can improve it—as well as make sure that you're the healthiest pear or apple on the tree.

those that are more difficult to break down and release glucose more slowly have a low GI. Slower rates of digestion, absorption, and glucose release also mean lower insulin levels (see www.glycemicindex.com).

You might be surprised to know that white bread, potatoes, and white rice all have a higher GI than chocolate. But it's important to keep in mind that the GI isn't a measure of how healthy a food is. For example, carrots and mangoes are better for you than angel food cake despite the fact that they have a higher GI.

Lisa had previously been eating a lot of low-calorie but high-GI foods, like 100-calorie snack packs of pretzels. Now she started thinking less in terms of calories and more in terms of whether the food was meeting her nutritional needs and whether it would cause a spike in her insulin levels. That was a big shift, but one she needed to make not only for her belly fat but also for her overall health. Relying on the calorie count alone to choose what to eat can perpetuate the idea that it's okay to eat low-calorie nutritionally empty junk—a practice that will make you fat, ill, and bloated. Counting calories instead of paying attention to the nutritional merits of the food you're eating is a practice based on fraudulent science. You should be thinking about how the food you eat can nourish and sustain you, not how many calories it has.

Lisa's belly fat never went away completely, but it did go down significantly. And there was more good news: she was able to stop her medications and control her diabetes with diet alone. Finally, instead of just going running, she started doing more core exercises and resistance training using light weights, which helped to strengthen her abdominal muscles and reduced her waistline.

11

Could It Be Celiac?

THESE DAYS IT SEEMS LIKE EVERYONE IS ON A GLUTEN-FREE DIET, AND chances are you know someone who's been diagnosed with celiac disease, is gluten sensitive, or has an allergy to wheat. The distinctions among these various conditions can be tricky, even for those of us in the medical community who diagnose and treat gluten-related disorders every day. If you're bloated or have ever wondered whether there might be a connection between what you're eating and how you're feeling, this chapter will help you figure out whether gluten might be that missing link.

Getting the Diagnosis Right

Jenny didn't have much in the way of bowel symptoms, just bloating after meals and some constipation. She came in to see me because of severe fatigue, brain fog, thinning hair, and a history of infertility, and she wanted advice on what supplements might be helpful for these problems. As soon as I heard her rattle off this list of seemingly unrelated symptoms, however, I suspected an underlying autoimmune disease. Autoimmune diseases tend to travel in packs, since whatever is stimulating the immune system likely affects multiple organs. I have lots of patients with autoimmune combinations like diabetes and psoriasis, or Crohn's and multiple sclerosis, or hypothyroidism and rheumatoid arthritis.

Jenny's blood work came back showing slightly abnormal thyroid function consistent with an underactive thyroid, which could definitely explain some of her symptoms. So I sent her to my local go-to thyroid expert. He checked some additional labs that confirmed hypothyroidism and started her on a low dose of thyroid hormone replacement therapy.

Jenny perked up a little on this regimen and her bowel movements became a bit more regular, but she still didn't feel quite right. We gave it another three months and rechecked her thyroid hormone levels. Everything was now perfectly in range, and she was tolerating the medication without any side effects. There was only one problem: she still didn't feel well. I believed Jenny when she said she was bone-tired. She looked fatigued just walking from the waiting room to the exam room, and she described feeling "out of it" at work.

A slightly low iron level was what ultimately tipped me off to what might be going on. Further testing revealed mild anemia, low vitamin D, and low magnesium. With so many different nutrients affected, malabsorption was now high on the list of culprits. I sent off a test for celiac disease I commonly use that checks for three different antibodies (anti-tissue transglutaminase, endomysial, and anti-gliadin), as well as two genetic subtypes associated with the disease (HLA-DQ2 and HLA-DQ8).

Jenny's test was strongly positive, with an estimated increased risk for celiac disease of thirty-one times higher than the general population. Since the prevalence of celiac disease in the United States is a little under 1 percent, her results were highly suggestive.

But I still didn't know for certain that Jenny had celiac disease. The blood test can predict risk, but without seeing the characteristic changes in her intestines, I couldn't be sure.

CELIAC DISEASE DEFINED

Celiac disease is an autoimmune digestive disorder that causes damage to the lining of the small intestine as a result of eating gluten, a protein found in wheat, rye, and barley. The symptoms vary tremendously, and lots of people are actually asymptomatic, that is, they have no symptoms.

Although you may only recently have heard of celiac disease, the foundation for the disease was laid down over ten thousand years ago when humans, previously nomadic hunter-gatherers, began to domesticate crops, introducing gluten into the diet for the first time. As early as the first century, a syndrome causing malabsorption and chronic diarrhea was described by the Greek physician Aretaeus of Cappadocia and given the name coeliac, from the Greek meaning "abdominal." In the 1880s, British physicians attributed chronic indigestion in some people to their diet, but they still didn't know what specifically was causing their symptoms. After the Second World War, the death rate in children with celiac disease plummeted from 35 percent to zero in conjunction with a shortage of bread, leading to the identification of gluten as the trigger for the disease.

DIAGNOSING CELIAC DISEASE

Celiac disease would certainly explain all of Jenny's symptoms. Now I needed to see if she had it. There are a couple of ways to examine the lining of the small intestine to check for the changes of celiac disease. Video capsule endoscopy, which entails swallowing a small capsule containing a camera that takes multiple pictures of the digestive tract as it travels from the mouth to the anus, can demonstrate the abnormalities. So can an upper endoscopy, which allows me to take biopsies of the lining that can be examined under the microscope to confirm the two characteristic findings: flattening of the fingerlike projections of the small intestine called villi that are designed to pull nutrients from digested matter as it passes through the GI tract and send them to the rest of the body, and an increase in white blood cells called lymphocytes, signaling the body's alerted immune response.

Jenny's biopsies had both findings. And yet another piece of the puzzle fell into place with this diagnosis. Jenny had mentioned she'd had a stress fracture while skiing the previous winter, and a bone density study had shown osteoporosis. At the time, this diagnosis was a surprise, since she was only thirty-two and not in the age group most at risk. Now it all made perfect sense: osteoporosis is strongly linked with celiac disease because of poor calcium absorption.

When I diagnose someone with celiac disease, I usually regard it as good news. Typically the patient, like Jenny, has been suffering for years with no answers as to why he or she feels so poorly and is in deteriorating health. When the diagnosis is finally made, it can feel like a light at the end of the tunnel, as well as validation that the symptoms are real—something that doctors along the way may have doubted. Best of all, celiac disease is treated by simply removing gluten from the diet. Occasionally someone has symptoms that don't improve despite eliminating gluten from the diet, and prescription medications have to be used, but that's rare.

So Jenny was relieved, but she was also perplexed. She felt poorly all the time, not just when she ate wheat, rye, or barley. I explained that over time, as a result of frequent exposure to gluten, the villi become flattened and are unable to absorb nutrients properly, especially those absorbed in the upper part of the small intestine, nutrients such as iron, magnesium, calcium, and the fat-soluble vitamins A, D, E, and K. When substances aren't properly absorbed, there can also be additional fermentation by bacteria, leading to bloating and diarrhea—although constipation like Jenny was experiencing can also occur.

Jenny had questions about medications, diet, pregnancy, and whether having celiac put her at risk for any cancers. I assured her that although there was a slightly higher incidence of lymphoma of the small bowel in untreated celiac disease, people in remission on a gluten-free diet (GFD) had no increased risk over the general population. There was more good news: the need for any medication to treat the disease was extremely low, and there was a good chance her infertility was a result of her celiac disease, which meant it would likely respond to the diet. Her thyroid condition, which had been diagnosed as Hashimoto's thyroiditis, was likely also related, since autoimmune thyroid diseases like Grave's and Hashimoto's are more common in people with celiac disease. The damage to the small intestine lining in celiac disease increases permeability in the gut, allowing toxic particles to gain access to the bloodstream and trigger an immune response in different organs, including the thyroid gland. People with the combination of celiac and thyroid disease are often able to treat both conditions through elimination of gluten. Jenny wasn't suffering from multiple different ailments; her problems were all related to the effect of gluten on various parts of her body. And chances were that all of them would be improved by getting rid of gluten.

Conditions Related to Celiac Disease

- Anemia
- Arthritis
- Ataxia
- Cancer (non-Hodgkin's lymphoma)
- Dermatitis
- Diabetes
- Infertility
- Irritable bowel syndrome (IBS)
- Lactose intolerance
- Liver disease
- Lymphocytic colitis or gastritis
- Migraines
- Peripheral neuropathy
- Obesity
- Osteoporosis
- Pancreatic disorders
- Thyroid disorders

Eating Gluten-Free

We spent most of Jenny's follow-up visit talking about her diet. Avoiding wheat, rye, and barley may sound pretty straightforward, but if you eat out frequently or buy prepared or packaged foods, it can be a big adjustment. Wheat is used as filler in lots of foods, and barley is often used as a sweetener, so you have to read labels carefully. My advice to Jenny was to stick to foods that didn't have an ingredient list: fruits, vegetables, nuts, seeds, eggs, potatoes, beans, yams, meat, poultry, fish, and shellfish. This was a great opportunity for her to eat "close to the ground" by avoiding packaged processed foods, and to discover some new grains.

In addition to brown rice, which she already ate a lot of, there was quinoa, cornmeal, amaranth, millet, and buckwheat. Oats can be problematic as they're often processed in facilities that also process wheat, barley, and rye, so there may be contamination with gluten, but in my experience most people with celiac disease have no problem tolerating oats that are certified gluten-free.

The one trap I asked her to be sure to avoid was consuming a lot of gluten-free but nutritionally empty foods like cookies, cakes, crackers, breakfast cereal, pancakes, bread, and pizza. Celiac disease developed because of the introduction of refined grains into our diet that our small intestines can't digest. Gluten-free junk is still junk, and swapping one refined grain for another can only lead to trouble down the road. People with celiac disease who eat a lot of gluten-free versions of foods that would normally have gluten in them, like pasta, cookies, bread, and pastries, generally have a much less robust response to their GFD. I encouraged Jenny to think about the fact that this disease was actually forcing her to behave in a way that conferred a real survival advantage: she would have to think about what she was eating, plan her meals carefully, avoid processed packaged foods, and cook more.

Jenny's story had a very happy ending. Excited about the diet and the prospect of feeling better, she plunged right in. But a month after starting the diet, she came to see me quite discouraged. She hadn't noticed any difference at all in her symptoms and was worried that the diagnosis was incorrect. She had been so hopeful that a GFD was the answer. I reassured her that it could take several months for the changes in her small intestine to normalize and her symptoms to improve. Eight months later when I saw her again, she was off her thyroid medication, much less fatigued, with regular bowel movements, a full head of hair, and negative celiac antibodies on her blood test. Her bloating was gone but she still had a bulging midsection—she was five months pregnant!

Is It Celiac Disease, Gluten Sensitivity, or Wheat Allergy?

The difference between celiac disease, gluten sensitivity, and a wheat allergy can be confusing. Our knowledge of these conditions and the science behind them is changing rapidly, but for now, this is what we know: celiac disease is an autoimmune disorder, caused by gluten, that occurs more in people who are genetically predisposed. There may be a variety of symptoms, including bloating, abdominal pain, diarrhea, a change in weight, constipation, fatigue, anemia, rashes, joint pain, neurological symptoms, a "foggy brain," other autoimmune phenomena, or no symptoms at all.

Gluten sensitivity (sometimes called non-celiac gluten sensitivity or gluten intolerance) can cause similar symptoms to celiac disease, but it isn't considered an autoimmune disorder and there is no damage to the lining of the small intestine. If you imagine a spectrum from normal to

Signs and Symptoms Associated with Celiac Disease

- Abdominal pain
- Arthritis
- Brain fog
- Bloating
- Bruising
- Constipation
- Depression
- Diarrhea
- Fatigue
- Fluid retention
- Gas
- Gastrointestinal bleeding
- Hair loss
- Infertility
- Iron deficiency
- Joint pain
- Menstrual abnormalities
- Mouth sores
- Muscle weakness/wasting
- Nausea
- Oily stools
- Osteoporosis
- Poor appetite
- Rashes (dermatitis herpetiformis)
- Stunted growth
- Tingling in extremities (neuropathy)
- Vertigo
- Vitamin deficiencies
- Vomiting
- Weight loss
- Weight gain

severe celiac disease, then gluten sensitivity is somewhere in the middle. The diagnosis is made on clinical grounds based on the response to withdrawing gluten from the diet, or reproducing symptoms by reintroducing it, although recent studies have shown that some gluten-sensitive patients may also have positive anti-gliadin antibodies. In addition to bloating and gas, manifestations outside the GI tract, such as rashes, brain fog, behavioral changes, joint pain, and fatigue, are extremely common with gluten sensitivity. Although there's no specific blood test or biopsy to diagnose it, it's estimated that many more people have gluten sensitivity than celiac disease.

A wheat allergy is a fairly common food allergy in children. It's when the immune system reacts to wheat by making immunoglobulin E antibodies, which can be measured by a blood test. It can also be diagnosed by injecting wheat under the skin. Bumps, redness, and irritation that occur within about fifteen minutes signify a positive test. Not everyone with a wheat allergy will have symptoms when they eat wheat.

The most common question from people diagnosed with a gluten-related disorder is whether they need to completely avoid gluten. It depends. If you have celiac disease, the answer is yes. Even if you're completely asymptomatic, ongoing exposure to gluten can cause progressive damage to your small intestine, increasing your chances of developing cancer and other related conditions and making it more likely that you'll eventually develop symptoms.

If you have gluten sensitivity, your symptoms should be your guide. Many of my patients tolerate inadvertently ingesting a bit of gluten or even plan to indulge from time to time, knowing they'll have symptoms. We don't think that eating a small amount of gluten in this setting results in any permanent damage to the lining of the small bowel or any other organs, although some researchers have raised concerns about neurological damage in gluten-sensitive people who continue to be exposed. For most people who are gluten-sensitive, once they eliminate gluten, they feel so much better that they can't be persuaded to reintroduce it.

If you have a wheat allergy and experience symptoms when you eat wheat, then you should avoid it. If you don't experience symptoms, then you can have it.

Some people discover they're gluten-sensitive while experimenting with low-carb diets that exclude most grains, including wheat, rye, and barley. Not only do a lot of them lose weight, but their bloating disappears and they feel better. So should we all be gluten-free? William Davis, MD, author of the widely popular and well-researched book *Wheat Belly*, suggests we should. The wheat we eat today is triticum wheat, which is very different from the einkorn wheat our forefathers ate, and that's a large part of why we're seeing such a rapid rise in the number of people who react to it.

In 1970 Norman Borlaug, PhD, won the Nobel Peace Prize for his techniques of hybridizing and crossbreeding wheat to increase the yield and decrease production costs, which was highly touted as a means to end world hunger. High-yield dwarf wheat now represents 99 percent of all the wheat consumed worldwide (although lots of people are still starving and many of us who aren't are overfed and undernourished). Dr. Davis suggests that this genetic tinkering has resulted in a product that has contributed more to our current obesity and diabetes epidemic than any other food. The fact is that today's wheat products raise blood sugar more than table sugar, ice cream, or a candy bar. It explains why so many people with celiac disease have weight gain, rather than the weight loss one would expect with malabsorption, and why so many others lose weight when they adopt a gluten-free lifestyle.

My own experience with gluten came in the form of brain fog and fatigue so intense that I had to pull over to the side of the road if I was driving. Like clockwork, the symptoms would occur about an hour after eating a high-gluten meal. A bagel was the worst; gluten-containing soy sauce and other mild exposure wasn't a problem.

At first I thought the symptoms must be a result of fluctuating blood sugar from eating foods that were releasing a lot of sugar into my bloodstream or from being hungry. But while I had no reactions to chocolate, large helpings of ice cream, or twenty-four-hour fasts, a slice of toast would leave me feeling awful. Weight gain was also part of my symptom complex, and I found that I could easily gain four to five pounds over just a few days when I was eating lots of wheat products. As is the case with many people, I wasn't able to truly appreciate my reaction until I completely eliminated gluten for a few weeks and then reintroduced it. It took several months of experimenting to realize that there was a clear correlation with gluten.

Neurological symptoms that include brain fog, headaches, and tingling in the extremities are common with both gluten sensitivity and celiac disease. Anxiety, depression, and even epilepsy have been described, and there is accumulating evidence to suggest that bipolar disorder and schizophrenia may also be exacerbated by gluten in some individuals.

I've had patients with completely unrelated conditions like diverticulosis describe dramatic improvements in their bloating after starting a GFD. These days, I recommend a GFD to my patients with inflammatory bowel diseases like Crohn's and ulcerative colitis for the simple reason that most of them have significant improvements in their inflammation and symptoms when they remove gluten from their diet. For irritable bowel syndrome (IBS), testing for celiac disease and a trial of a GFD is a must, even if the test is negative, since many IBS sufferers actually have undiagnosed celiac disease or gluten sensitivity. Acid reflux, chronic constipation, and microscopic colitis may all potentially improve with a GFD. Celiac disease and gluten sensitivity aside, the condition I see responding the most to a GFD is bloating from various different causes.

I have to admit that up until a few years ago, I was like many doctors who scoff at the idea of a gluten-free diet for someone who doesn't have celiac disease. But after seeing so many patients experience improvements in their bloating, GI distress, and overall sense of well-being, I'm a believer in giving a GFD a try if you have GI symptoms. Not everyone will feel better, but there's not much of a downside to avoiding gluten for a few weeks, and the benefits may be substantial. Try my Gutbliss Plan for just ten days (see Chapter 23) to see if you could be one of the millions of people whose life is changed by eliminating gluten.

12

Is There an Inflammation Connection?

WHEN IT COMES TO YOUR DIGESTIVE TRACT, IT CAN BE HARD TO PIN-point exactly what's making you sick, but bloating is never a "normal" occurrence; it's always a sign that something isn't quite right in your gut.

Inflammation is our body's response to harmful stimuli, and a protective attempt to stop injury and heal tissue. Long-standing, low-grade inflammation seems to be the root cause behind many conditions, from Crohn's to coronary artery disease. Because our environment and much of our food contain so many harmful chemicals, living with inflammation has become a way of life for many people.

There's a particular type of intestinal inflammation that primarily affects middle-aged women and can cause significant bloating. We're still learning about what causes it and how it can be improved, but, as in other types of inflammation, what you put into your body plays a huge role. The good news is that if you have it, there's a lot you can do to help yourself feel better.

Biopsies: A Key Tool for Solving GI Mysteries

If you have bloating and a change in bowel habits and are having a colonoscopy, it's important that biopsies be taken from throughout your colon, including the top, bottom, and middle parts. Inflammation isn't always visible to the naked eye, and it can be patchy and missed if enough areas aren't sampled. I've encountered lots of people who've suffered from bloating and loose stools and who were told, after a "normal" colonoscopy, that it was all stress-related, only to have the procedure repeated years later with biopsies that find significant inflammation.

"Why Do I Feel Awful?"

Mary was referred to me for diarrhea, nausea, and terrible bloating. Initial stool studies and labs were normal and, because of the severity of her symptoms, a colonoscopy was the next step. Surprisingly, Mary's colon looked completely normal: no ulcerations to suggest inflammation from ulcerative colitis or Crohn's disease, no infected pockets consistent with diverticulitis, and no redness hinting at a recent infection. I took multiple random biopsies throughout the colon, each one about the size of the head of a pin. I was looking for microscopic inflammation: changes in the surface lining that aren't visible to the naked eye but show up under the microscope and could be the cause of Mary's symptoms.

Mary's biopsies did indeed reveal inflammation—a condition called collagenous colitis, which is a type of microscopic colitis visible only under the microscope. In Mary's case, the inflammation had produced a thick band of connective tissue called collagen under the surface of the colon lining that was preventing proper absorption, resulting in bloating and loose stools. We're not sure what's responsible for this type of microscopic inflammation, but it may be related to long-standing irritation of the lining by various substances. The immune system seems to be responding to something in the gut that's not supposed to be there, and the end result is inflammation.

Understanding Microscopic Colitis

Microscopic colitis is different from ulcerative colitis (UC) and Crohn's disease (CD), two forms of inflammatory bowel diseases (IBD) that cause inflammation in the digestive tract that you can see with the naked eye. UC affects the colon. CD can affect any part of the GI tract but occurs most commonly in the small intestine. With IBD you can see lots of different manifestations of inflammation in the gut—ulceration and bleeding in the lining, as well as thickening and narrowing in some parts of the bowels. UC and CD usually cause symptoms that are more severe than microscopic colitis, and there can be associated symptoms outside the intestines, like fever, kidney stones, skin lesions, and ulcers in the mouth, which don't occur with microscopic colitis, although they can all cause fatigue and joint pain. Unlike IBD, microscopic colitis doesn't lead to cancer and rarely requires surgical intervention. Although IBD and microscopic colitis are distinct clinical conditions, they're both autoimmune diseases, where the body is reacting to an unknown stimulus. Almost half of all patients with microscopic colitis and many patients with IBD have a concomitant autoimmune disorder like thyroid or celiac disease.

We used to think microscopic colitis was rare—probably because too often we didn't take biopsies when the colon looked normal—but recent studies show that it can be the cause in up to 13 percent of people with unexplained diarrhea and bloating. Most people with microscopic colitis report five or more watery, non-bloody stools daily, almost always associated with bloating. The symptoms can wax and wane—some of my patients will have no symptoms for months at a time and then have flare-ups that last just as long. Fortunately, most people respond well to identifying and eliminating triggers, although some require medical therapy.

We don't know what causes collagenous colitis, but we do know what makes it worse. Common dietary triggers include dairy, caffeine, and artificial sweeteners. There's also a strong association with gluten in some people. A wide variety of medications have been associated with microscopic colitis, including nonsteroidal anti-inflammatory drugs (NSAIDs), aspirin, certain kinds of antidepressants (selective serotonin reuptake inhibitors or SSRIs), acid-suppressive drugs (proton pump inhibitors), and cholesterol-lowering agents (statins). In my patients with microscopic colitis, a history of taking NSAIDs is the most frequently reported factor associated with symptoms.

Collagenous colitis is most common in middle-aged women, although it can occur in men and women of any age. There's another form of microscopic colitis called lymphocytic colitis, which has identical symptoms to collagenous colitis and is also not visible to the naked eye, but instead of a collagen band there is an abundance of white blood cells called lymphocytes in the lining. In both collagenous colitis and lymphocytic colitis, the colon looks normal when it's inspected at colonoscopy, and the diagnosis is only made when biopsies are taken and examined.

TREATMENT STRATEGIES

When we're not quite sure what causes a condition, there tends to be a lot of trial and error in the treatment. With microscopic colitis, we use everything but the kitchen sink: Pepto-Bismol, antidiarrheals, antibiotics, salicylic acid derivatives related to aspirin but with the opposite effect, bile-salt binders, steroids, and more potent immune-suppressing drugs. The wide range of unrelated therapies suggests that we're still stumbling around in the dark a little in terms of both what causes the inflammation and how to make it better. One thing we look at very closely, however, is the person's diet and how it may be triggering symptoms.

Mary was taking NSAIDs and antidepressants, both of which are associated with microscopic colitis, but even more striking were her dietary risk factors. Although her condition was much improved compared to how it had been when she was in her early twenties, at fifty-five Mary was still suffering from an eating disorder. Her diet was rigid and restrictive: lots of yogurt, cottage cheese, coffee, sugar-free candy, and diet soda, and very few fruits or vegetables. Everything she ate was artificially sweetened, and none of it seemed particularly nutritious. She was consuming ten packs of sugar-free chewing gum a day, which for some people with eating disorders can be a tactic to avoid eating real food, keeping the jaws busy but the stomach empty.

I thought Mary would be thrilled to finally have a solid diagnosis and to hear the good news that this was something we could treat by changing her diet, as well as switching around some medications. Instead, she burst into tears. "You're taking all my food away," she sobbed. She had been eating like this for a long time, and the idea of venturing out and eating things not on her approved food list was very scary.

I reminded her that there were lots of other foods besides dairy, caffeine, and low-calorie sweeteners that would be safe for her to eat. "But I don't eat those things," she told me. "I eat cottage cheese and yogurt and coffee and soda. I *can't* eat those other things."

For someone like Mary, who'd been battling an eating disorder for decades, I can only imagine how intimidating and overwhelming all of these dietary changes coming at once must have felt like. The small cache of foods she was eating every day was her safety net, and I was yanking it out from under her. But Mary's body was speaking to her, and she couldn't continue not to listen. Her immune system was reacting to something, and her poor, inflamed colon was bearing the brunt of it. We finally knew what was going on; now we needed to figure out what to do about it.

I enlisted the help of Elise Museles, an integrative nutritionist whose practical approach to food can whip any pantry into shape. Elise focuses on helping people to get organized in the kitchen with menu planning, batch cooking, and also focuses on the psychology of eating.

I explained Mary's circumstances to Elise and what we were looking to eliminate, at least for a trial period of four to six weeks to assess her response. It also seemed like a great time to begin a gentle conversation with Mary about incorporating more nutrient-rich food into her diet.

THE CHALLENGE OF CHANGE

Changing our food habits can be a little threatening for all of us, not just someone with an eating disorder. Most of us eat the same thirty or so foods in rotation, our shopping carts and dinner plates looking virtually the same from one week to the next. We might have a little more melon in June and a bit more squash in September, but the basics tend to remain constant. We usually think we're eating more broadly than we are, but when we break down the ingredients, it tends to be the same procession of wheat, corn, and dairy in various guises—foods that aren't exactly nutrition powerhouses. Variety is a hugely important aspect of nutrition because different foods have different nutrients and the more of them we eat, the healthier we are.

Mary wasn't doing the Big Four particularly well, which may have been, at least in part, why she had developed inflammation. If you think of microscopic colitis not as a complicated autoimmune disorder but as a simple matter of what the digestive tract likes and doesn't like, and you look at some of the things it reacts to, a pattern starts to emerge:

- More than half the world's population can't digest dairy properly.
- Caffeine increases acid production, irritates the lining of the GI tract, and can cause diarrhea.
- Artificial sweeteners are artificial substances (I really have a hard time calling them foods) that can't be properly broken down and absorbed by the intestines.
- NSAIDs and aspirin can damage the protective mucus and bicarbonate layers of the GI tract.
- Proton pump inhibitors change the pH of the GI tract, making it less able to absorb nutrients and more hospitable to invading bacteria.

It makes sense that these substances might contribute to inflammation, and to avoid them if your digestive tract is already inflamed. Recent studies also show a strong association between microscopic colitis and gluten: as many as 15 percent of people diagnosed with microscopic colitis also have celiac disease, so it's important to screen for it with a blood test or biopsies of the small intestine. Lots of my patients successfully get their colitis symptoms under control with a gluten-free diet even without a formal diagnosis of celiac disease, raising the possibility that modern-day wheat is also something the gut doesn't like.

GUT FEELINGS: STRONG YET SENSITIVE

The gut is such a complex and sensitive organ that we don't know all the details of what causes it to become inflamed. One thing we do know is that most of the body's lymphoid tissue is located in the GI tract—an area that, spread out, would cover an entire football field! That's a lot of surface area through which invading toxins, bacteria, and viruses can gain access. The gut has special tissue (gut-associated lymphoid tissue, or GALT) that protects the body from invasion by fencing off potential toxins and other harmful substances and preventing them from entering the bloodstream. White blood cells are the soldiers of the immune system, carrying out attacks and defending against foreign invaders.

Other factors that help the gut immune system keep us healthy include a low pH that kills unwelcome bacteria, mucus that can neutralize organisms, potent detoxifying enzymes in saliva and bile, and hordes of good bacteria. When the system is working well, it can protect us from highly poisonous substances. When it's not, minor insults can become major problems. Why not support this amazing terrain within by protecting it as it protects us? And how fortunate that the foods we eat can have a direct healing effect.

Two months after her diagnosis, I was excited to meet with Mary and hear how she was doing. She'd seen both Elise and her therapist a few times and had summoned the courage to make some big changes. She'd gotten rid of most of the gum, diet soda, dairy, and caffeine. Her diet was still pretty limited, but she was making steel-cut oatmeal with nuts and berries for breakfast and eating salads for lunch most days. Dinner tended to be cereal with almond milk or chicken with rice. Other than an occasional soft stool once a week, her bowels were back to normal and her bloating was almost completely gone.

I was fortunate to be able to diagnose Mary and witness a real improvement in her symptoms. So many of the patients I see these days have vague, nonspecific, poorly defined symptoms that are difficult to nail down and even more difficult to treat. I can't always make a specific diagnosis, but I frequently have a strong sense that many of them are being slowly poisoned. And when I look at their GI tracts and see the high prevalence of inflammation, my sense of unease is confirmed.

Our food comes with lots and lots of chemicals these days, and keeping them out of the GI tract is increasingly challenging for all of us. If you have an inflammatory condition, however, it's essential that you examine your diet and look for potential triggers. As Mary's story makes clear, sometimes the foods we rely on most are the ones predisposing us to pain and illness. Taking a close look at what you're eating and resolving to break bad food habits can be challenging and scary, but it may be the most important step you take on the road to healing inflammation and finding your gutbliss.

13

What About IBS?

WE KNOW VERY LITTLE ABOUT WHAT CAUSES IRRITABLE BOWEL SYN-drome (IBS) and how to treat it, but 15 to 20 percent of Americans suffer from it, and it can have a profoundly negative effect on their quality of life. IBS treatment costs billions in both direct costs such as prescriptions and over-the-counter medications and indirect costs such as absenteeism from work and lost productivity. Perhaps the most significant cost of IBS is the intangible expense of a decreased quality of life to the individual. It's the most common diagnosis made by gastroenterologists, yet the one we know the least about.

IBS involves abdominal pain or discomfort that's usually associated with constipation, diarrhea, or both, and virtually everyone complains of bloating. That's the *what*. In this chapter we'll explore the *why*, as well as my recommendations on how to approach this puzzling, poorly defined, and frequently debilitating diagnosis.

Mind/Body Breakthrough

In 1975 Harvard cardiologist Herbert Benson, MD, wrote a book called *The Relaxation Response*. His simple observation that blood pressure was higher in the doctor's office than when patients measured it themselves at home caused him to speculate that there might be a connection between stress and high blood pressure. Ridiculed by his colleagues, he took his theory to the lab. He taught monkeys to control their blood pressure with a reward system that used colored lights, eventually training them to lower their blood pressure with just their thoughts when the appropriate lights were turned on. He next turned to transcendental meditation (TM), ultimately proving that TM alone could lead to startling changes in heart rate, metabolic rate, and breathing rate and that as a group, people who practiced TM had much lower blood pressure. Of course, practitioners of Eastern medicine had known about these techniques and used them in their practice for hundreds of years, but Dr. Benson's results were groundbreaking in Western medicine, introducing the concept that the mind and the body were not separate systems that functioned independently.

It's obvious to most of us that the brain is connected to the rest of the body. When you decide to go for a run or to pick up the phone, your brain sends a message to the appropriate muscles for the activity to be carried out. That's easy to understand when we're talking about actionable things like moving your hands and feet. But what about how your body responds to emotions?

Here's the example I like to use when I'm trying to explain that what's in your head is also in your body: you're walking through the woods and a bear jumps out at you.

How do you respond? Your adrenal glands send hormones coursing through your body, including adrenaline and cortisol, mediators of the fight-or-flight response that provides us with quick bursts of energy to face down a predator or run for cover. These hormones cause a cascade of changes that occur almost immediately: your heart rate increases, you start to breathe fast, you get sweaty, the hair on your body stands on end, your blood pressure goes up, and your pupils dilate. As Dr. Benson suspected, emotions such as fear and stress result in real and measurable changes. These feelings aren't just in your mind; they're also very much in your body, especially your gut.

Stuck in Overdrive

Our adrenal system has evolved powerfully to protect our survival. In times of stress or threat, it diverts resources from systems such as the digestive tract, so that all energy and attention can be focused on the stressor at hand. Then, once the danger passes, the relaxation response kicks in, allowing everything to get back to a normal, mellow state. But modern life tends to keep many of us constantly revved up. Our body experiences this as an onslaught of one stressor after another. Being in a chronic fight-or-flight, stressed-out state can have devastating effects on the body. It impairs our ability to think clearly; decreases thyroid function, immunity, and bone density; and increases blood pressure, blood sugar, and inflammation. It accelerates the aging process so we don't just feel stressed out, we look it, too. Stress even affects weight distribution, increasing deposition of the dreaded belly fat that's associated with metabolic syndrome and a higher chance of dying sooner rather than later.

Stress and IBS: Is There a Connection?

Of all the things that conspire to cause GI problems, it's been my observation that stress is both the most prevalent and the most dangerous.

Like many of my patients, you may have a lot of stress in your life. You may also have been diagnosed with IBS. But could stress actually be causing your IBS? The answer is: we don't know. There definitely seems to be a cohort of people whose symptoms are entirely due to stress, but more commonly stress is an exacerbating factor, making symptoms worse. In fact, stress doesn't just contribute to IBS; it's a hugely important aspect of practically every chronic disease, including cancer, arthritis, gout, heart disease, diabetes, and countless others.

Chances are you've had the sensation of butterflies in your stomach, nausea, or feeling like you have to move your bowels right before a big event. Stress really wreaks havoc on your digestive system: it increases stomach acid production, causing heartburn and nausea; shunts blood away from the intestines, interfering with digestion and absorption of nutrients; decreases enzyme secretion; slows down stomach emptying; and speeds up colonic contractions—all of which can add up to some serious bloating.

Stress also induces responses in the gut that can affect your immune system, including increased intestinal permeability associated with leaky gut and food allergies, greater susceptibility to inflammation and infection, and alterations in the ratio of beneficial to harmful bacteria.

Gut-directed hypnotherapy (GHT) to relieve stress has been found to be an effective therapy for IBS in a number of studies, and superior to medical treatment alone. Quality-of-life outcomes are improved and GHT has a long-term positive effect, even in difficult-to-treat cases of IBS.

Stress and Medical Bias

Not only can stress affect how you feel, but it can also influence how you are diagnosed and treated. When people appear anxious and stressed during medical appointments, it can be distracting for the physician, who may then surmise, incorrectly, that stress and anxiety are the only problems at hand. This error happens far more frequently with women patients. Even today, the ancient bias toward relegating symptoms and disease in women to "hysteria" (a term rooted in the Greek word for uterus) remains a huge problem. I've seen women suffer needlessly and doubt their own intuition about their bodies because their complaints are incorrectly attributed purely to stress. They're dismissed with a pat on the head and an admonition to reduce their stress instead of a more thoughtful and comprehensive diagnosis and treatment plan—which, of course, might include stress reduction.

A Different Way to Look at IBS

Controlling your stress can be a huge part of getting your IBS symptoms under control, but it may not be the only thing you need to do. If stress alone isn't causing your IBS, what else might be involved?

One of the classic experiments to investigate the cause of IBS involved inflating a balloon in the rectum. People with IBS felt discomfort at a much lower volume of balloon distention compared to people without

Signs and Symptoms of Stress

If you think stress may be contributing to your GI symptoms but you're not sure, here are some useful signs and symptoms to look for:

Physical Symptoms
- Stiff or tense muscles, especially in the neck or shoulders
- Headaches
- Shakiness or tremors
- Loss of interest in sex
- Weight gain or loss
- Restlessness

Behavioral Symptoms
- Procrastination
- Grinding teeth
- Difficulty completing work assignments
- Changes in the amount of alcohol or food you consume
- Sleeping too much or too little

Emotional Symptoms
- Crying
- Overwhelming sense of tension or pressure
- Trouble relaxing
- Nervousness
- Quick temper
- Depression
- Poor concentration
- Trouble remembering things
- Loss of sense of humor

IBS. This observation was the basis for the theory of visceral hypersensitivity, which concluded that people with IBS have a lower-than-normal threshold for discomfort with stretching and distention of hollow organs like the intestines. Other proposed theories include low-grade inflammation that you can't readily see on endoscopy, and alterations in the way the gut and the brain communicate through the millions of nerve cells located in the GI tract that have sometimes been called "the second brain."

The problem with these theories is that they tell us *what* may be happening, but they don't tell us *why*. *Why* do some people feel uncomfortable when their intestines have even small amounts of stool or gas in them? *Why* do biopsies of the colon sometimes show chronic nonspecific inflammation under the microscope, despite a normal colonoscopy? *Why* are the gut and the brain not communicating properly? *Why* is your bowel irritable?

IBS is frequently referred to as a diagnosis of exclusion: your doctor can't find anything else wrong; therefore, it must be IBS. But if you slice up the IBS pie and take a good look, you actually find lots of potential explanations for what might be causing your symptoms (see "Potential Causes of IBS Symptoms," page 128): gluten sensitivity, parasites, bacterial overgrowth, leaky gut, and microscopic colitis. For every condition we know about, there are probably a hundred more we don't: viruses, allergies, and autoimmune problems that haven't been discovered yet. And there can be multiple things at play—a chronic infection causing food allergies, plus side effects from your antidepressant and a suboptimal diet.

For all of these reasons, I consider IBS a set of symptoms, the cause(s) of which can vary tremendously from person to person, rather than a definitive disease or diagnosis. It's sort of like fatigue—not a disease unto itself, but a symptom with hundreds of possible causes, no single test to diagnose it, and no unifying treatment. If I went to see a doctor because I felt tired, and she told me my diagnosis was fatigue and that the solution was to take pills for the rest of my life to pep me up, I would question her diagnosis and treatment. I'd want to know why I felt tired, what was causing it, and what I could do to resolve or improve it, besides taking medications.

IBS causes real symptoms and real suffering, and it's absolutely essential to figure out why, rather than just accept IBS as the diagnosis and resign yourself to a life of pharmaceutical intervention. Remember, IBS is a description of your symptoms (*your bowel is irritable*), not what's causing them (*Why is your bowel irritable?*).

Potential Causes of IBS Symptoms

- Aerophagia (air swallowing)
- Antibiotic use
- Bacterial overgrowth (dysbiosis)
- Bile acid malabsorption
- Bile gastritis
- Carbohydrate malabsorption
- Celiac disease
- Constipation
- Crohn's disease
- Diet
- Diverticulosis
- Eating disorders
- Eosinophilic gastroenteritis
- Food allergies
- Fructose malabsorption
- Gallbladder dysfunction
- Gallstones
- Gastroparesis
- Gluten sensitivity
- *Helicobacter pylori*
- Infections
- Lactose intolerance
- Leaky gut syndrome
- Liver disease
- Medication side effects
- Motility disorders
- Microscopic colitis
- Parasites (especially *Giardia* and *Blastocystis hominis*)
- Small intestinal bacterial overgrowth (SIBO)
- Stress
- Thyroid disorders
- Ulcerative colitis

Unknowns and Economics

Part of why people aren't getting the answers they need is because we don't necessarily have them to give. If you look up IBS, you'll find information on subtype classifications, diagnostic criteria, neural pathways, and abnormal processing and stimulation. You'll also read that most of the body's feel-good hormone, serotonin, is housed in the gut, where it acts as a neurotransmitter. What does this all mean? No one knows for sure, but what we do know is that there's a lot of money at stake.

Most IBS research is funded by the pharmaceutical industry. That doesn't automatically mean it's bad research, but it makes it a lot harder to tell if it's good research. The *Washington Post* reported recently that "as the drug industry's influence over research grows, so does the potential for bias," and a recent study from the University of Pennsylvania found that the odds of research coming to a conclusion favorable to a drug are 3.6 times greater when that research is funded by the company making the drug.

Serotonin in the gut has been the subject of intense pharmaceutical science. Companies have spent millions of dollars on research and millions more promoting drugs for IBS that reduce gut motility by blocking serotonin, and others that increase motility by increasing serotonin. Some of these drugs are helpful, although in my experience they don't completely ameliorate IBS symptoms, and they're often poorly tolerated due to side effects. Even when they do help, it still doesn't explain why you have abdominal pain, diarrhea, constipation, or altered motility in the first place.

I can't give you medical advice about what drug, if any, to take for your IBS, but I do recommend that you hold whatever you're considering taking—a prescription, an over-the-counter medication, a supplement, or an herbal remedy—to the same reasonable standard: it should make you feel better and not harm you.

The reality is that no two patients experience IBS in exactly the same way. What works for your friend may not work for you. Information from magazines and the Internet can be confusing—particularly when it's designed to sell you something. Some Web sites advise increasing soluble fiber; others say soluble fiber will make you worse, and memorizing lists of the ratio of soluble to insoluble fiber in fruits and vegetables is no easy feat. I've had people tell me about diluted apple cider vinegar cures, crushed papaya seeds and honey, energy healing, Chinese herbs, cod liver oil, vitamin D supplements, FODMAP diets, prescription antispasmodics, probiotics, aloe vera juice, flax seed smoothies, psyllium husk, juice cleansing, and dozens of other things that helped their symptoms.

Bottom line: What works best for IBS is what works for you. I'm a believer in the Hippocratic principle of primum non nocere—above all, do no harm—so I'm generally willing to consider most things as long as the benefit clearly outweighs the risk and there are tangible improvements.

In that spirit, let me tell you about some of my patients who were diagnosed with IBS and what's been helpful for them.

Mindy: When Stress Isn't the Whole Story

Mindy had a history of constipation dating back to childhood, much of it related to anxiety about using the bathroom at school or around strangers. She was on three different drugs for depression and two for anxiety. Over the years her constipation had gotten much worse, despite a healthy diet. She used to exercise a fair amount, but the psychiatric drugs had made her gain a lot of weight and she had become increasingly sedentary. She was feeling tired and slowed down, and so was her GI tract.

Mindy was taking huge doses of a stimulant laxative but moving her bowels only once a week, and she was bloated and uncomfortable all the time. Her colon had become dependent on the laxatives, so she couldn't have a bowel movement without them—a major problem with stimulant laxatives and the reason we caution against using them regularly—and she was requiring higher and higher doses. The process of getting the stool out was an ordeal. It was hard and impacted, and she often experienced bleeding and intense pain with bowel movements. On rectal exam she had a deep midline fissure, which is a tear in the delicate lining that can occur as a result of chronic constipation. She had a lot of difficulty relaxing her sphincter muscles, and I could feel them clamped like a vise around my finger on the rectal exam.

My first recommendation was to try to get her off some of the psychiatric drugs, which included a tricyclic antidepressant and a selective serotonin reuptake inhibitor (SSRI), both of which are known to cause constipation. Her psychiatrist agreed to stop the tricyclic and switch the SSRI to another brand, but neither change made any difference. We ended up decreasing the doses of all her medications, and within a few weeks her bowel regularity started to improve. I added my old-fashioned recommendations of a heating pad, soothing music, and abdominal self-massage with a two-pound dumbbell in a clockwise direction to help move the stool along. That helped, too.

Part of Mindy's problem was anismus: her pelvic muscles were tightening instead of relaxing during bowel movements, making it really difficult for the stool to come out. The longer it stayed in, the harder it got, so that by the time it finally made an appearance, it was like giving birth. Anticipating pain from her anal fissure, Mindy would delay having bowel movements if she felt the urge to go at work or anywhere outside of her house.

We see this problem in babies and toddlers a lot. They get dehydrated and constipated and then have a hard stool that's difficult to come out and causes a fissure. Subsequent bowel movements are painful because of the fissure, so they start to hold them in, leading to a vicious cycle of harder, more painful stools.

Getting the stool soft enough so it's easy to pass is part of the remedy, and that's exactly what we did with Mindy. I started her on a teaspoon of ground psyllium husk dissolved in a large glass of water three times a day for the first week, and then increased it to a heaping tablespoon with each meal. I persuaded her to dramatically increase her water consumption—a simple but supereffective way to soften the stool. She went from a total of two glasses of water a day to three glasses with each dose of psyllium.

The psyllium fiber supplement created a much stronger urge to go, but she still felt very bloated, and her stool was sometimes pasty and hard to push out. I added two capfuls of an osmotic cathartic at bedtime and told her that as the stool became easier to pass, she could cut the dose in half or skip it altogether. An osmotic cathartic works by drawing water into the stool to make it softer. Side effects can include diarrhea and gas. I'm not keen on the fact that the popular osmotic cathartics on the market are made with polyethylene glycol, which has a number of industrial uses that give one pause. My goal is always to have patients stop using it as soon as possible, or to limit it to emergency use when things get really backed up. But the fact is for many people the combination of fiber and an osmotic cathartic works really well. Fiber alone left Mindy feeling bloated: plugged with a bigger, bulkier plug. When we added the cathartic, things really started to move nicely.

The next step was weaning her off the stimulant laxatives. Over time her colon had developed a tolerance to these drugs, needing higher and higher amounts of them to do its work. It took us about four months of slowly lowering the dose before we could eventually stop them altogether. People who've used a lot of laxatives will often develop this kind of colonic inertia where things just stop moving, and the arduous process of retraining the colon can take months and in some cases even years.

To complicate things, Mindy had started getting weekly high-pressure colonics, and now her bowels were conditioned to sit back and wait for a jet hose to do their job. It was hard to get her to stop the colonics; she would feel agonizingly full of stool and knew that the colonics would provide instant relief. But she also knew that in the long term they were part of the problem, creating a dependency on alternative ways of emptying her colon. So she started weaning herself off those, too, increasing the interval between them from one week to two, then monthly and eventually none at all.

Mindy was finally starting to approach normalcy: a good-sized bowel movement every other day without bleeding or pain. But she was still tense and nervous, especially about bowel movements. She heavily favored using the toilet only at home, and it was still taking half an hour for her to have a bowel movement. It was time to pull out the really big guns: biofeedback practitioner extraordinaire Emily Perlman. After several sessions with Emily, Mindy started to catch on to the techniques of deep breathing and guided imagery. Not only did her sphincter start to unclench, but the smooth muscles throughout other parts of her body also started to relax, resulting in a healthy decrease in her blood pressure.

Mindy is still taking a fair number of drugs, not exercising regularly, and still wound pretty tight. But she's a lot better than she was. Not perfect, but not in pain and not uncomfortable all the time.

Leslie: Conquering "Crummy Diet Syndrome"

Leslie had terrible eating habits. She was a picky eater as a child, and her parents' response had been to let her eat whatever she wanted and avoid what she didn't. She was now in her twenties, and her palate was firmly set. Her food journal looked something like this: a bagel with cream cheese or an English muffin with jelly for breakfast, McDonald's chicken nuggets and fries for lunch, and pasta with butter for dinner, plus Gatorade or soda. Nothing else. No fruits or vegetables ever—she didn't like the taste or the texture. She was in her sixth year of college after spending a few semesters at home on the couch. She complained of frequent debilitating pain, constant bloating, and occasional vomiting.

Leslie had what I call crummy diet syndrome, which can be a lot more challenging to treat than other causes of IBS. She also had a vested interest in being sick, and that can be even harder to manage than IBS and crummy diet syndrome combined. At this point Leslie's GI problems had become her lifeboat: her rationale for why she couldn't get up early enough to make it to class, finish college, get a summer job, cook a meal, or clean her room. And she was clinging to it for dear life.

I'm not trying to make light of Leslie's situation, or anyone in a similar predicament. It's an absolutely paralyzing position to be in, and it's not that difficult to see how it can develop. When my eight-year-old has a sore throat and fever, she gets to stay home, sleep in, hang out in her pajamas all day, eat Popsicles, and watch movies with my husband or me. We're constantly rubbing her little head, cuddling her, and saying how sorry we are that she's under the weather. She normally likes school, but third grade can have a hard time competing with this kind of attention. If her recovery seems a little slow, sometimes I have to change up the strategy. Green veggie juices take the place of Popsicles, and workbooks replace movie watching. There may even be some medicinal room cleaning, which usually has a remarkable therapeutic effect. My daughter's go-slow recovery isn't malingering; it's human nature. And lots of coddling and sympathy when kids are sick isn't bad parenting. But it can leave some kids yearning for that feeling of suspended responsibility and being taken care of that can seductively follow them into adulthood. It may contribute to a persona that focuses on illness rather than health, where a diagnosis can become a crutch for avoiding life's challenges and responsibilities.

Sometimes patients may feel they have to exaggerate and embellish because otherwise they won't be taken seriously, especially with conditions like IBS, since, as mentioned, there's already a tendency on the part of the medical community to assume it's all in your head. Maybe Leslie really did have a rare, undiagnosed disorder that was responsible for her symptoms rather than just poor eating habits. Medicine is full of stories of people who have had rare conditions, were labeled hypochondriacs for decades, and then were finally vindicated when some expert diagnosed them. But for the purposes of this discussion, let's assume that what Leslie had was a daily stomachache from her nutrient-poor, overprocessed diet.

Leslie had been to multiple doctors. In conversations with me they all expressed the same skepticism about her symptoms, but never to Leslie or her family. Her remarkably poor eating habits were the elephant in the room—overwhelmingly present, but no one was talking about it. She'd had an expensive medical workup at two excellent clinics: upper endoscopy, colonoscopy, video capsule endoscopy, gastric emptying studies, small bowel barium exams, ultrasound, CAT (computerized axial tomography) scans of the abdomen and pelvis, gallbladder scans, tilt table studies, brain MRIs (magnetic resonance imagings), bile duct examinations, and multiple blood tests looking for everything from Lyme disease to cancer. She had tried a dozen different prescription medications without any improvement. By the time she came to me, there wasn't anything else to be done other than to have a frank conversation.

The first thing I said to Leslie was that I believed she really didn't feel well and was suffering, which was the truth. I also told her that there had been enough tests and that I didn't see the need to do any more. Instead, I focused on what we needed to do to improve things, and how much better her life would be when she felt well.

Rather than dwell on a name for her diagnosis or the science behind it, I simply referred to it as "her symptoms," and we found a therapist she liked whom she could discuss things with. After about a year she finally felt comfortable revealing a history of a restrictive eating disorder as a teen, which had never been acknowledged by her parents despite tremendous weight loss and social withdrawal. The cognitive behavioral therapy with the therapist was far more helpful than any of the IBS medications that had been tried in the past, although it was very slow progress.

I assured Leslie we would also be taking baby steps with her diet, focusing on what was missing rather than what she had to cut out. She made a pact with me to add one fruit, one vegetable, and one glass of water a day to her diet, and she agreed to take a probiotic to increase the amount of healthy bacteria in her colon. There were no other rules or restrictions.

She started with carrots, progressed to peas, and after about six months was experimenting with string beans and asparagus. She didn't mind blended fruit, so we started alternating her usual breakfast bagel with smoothies made with berries, bananas, and coconut milk. Chicken nuggets and fries were still in heavy rotation, but she was also working rotisserie chicken and baked sweet potatoes into the mix, and adding broccoli to her pasta. She surprised me by offering to go cold turkey on the Gatorade and soda if she could have sparkling water mixed with fruit juice instead.

Slowly but surely, things started to improve—she didn't look or feel as bloated, she stopped complaining about pain and vomiting, and her pasty complexion that had been prone to pimples started to clear up. I don't know whether she finished her degree or got a job because eventually she stopped coming to see me. But I did feel a shift with Leslie: an unspoken nod to the idea that things could be different, that she could be a little sick instead of a lot sick, and that her illness didn't need to define her so completely.

Carol: Keep Trying Until You Find What Works

Carol was already quite progressive in terms of food and fitness when she came to see me. She was a slim, trim vegetarian who knew a lot about nutrition and looked the part. But she didn't feel well. She had daily bloating and pain after almost everything she ate and had whittled her diet down to mostly tea, toast, and yogurt in an effort to find out whether her symptoms might be food related. But even with that restricted regimen, she still felt terrible. A bout of severe pain prompted a late-night visit to the emergency room, where an ultrasound of the abdomen and blood work were both normal. She was sent home with a prescription for acid suppression, which had no effect on her symptoms.

Carol ate a lot of fruit and vegetables, and no meat, poultry, fish, or eggs, but her diet was still quite high in fat. Her only animal protein was dairy and she ate a ton of it: Greek yogurt with berries for breakfast, cottage cheese and fruit for lunch, feta cheese on salad or pasta in a heavy cream sauce for dinner. Her snacks were cheese and crackers, potato chips, or buttered popcorn. Most nights she had a glass or two of wine, although not recently, given how sick she was feeling.

Carol had been tested for celiac disease in the past and the results had been negative. She'd tried cutting back on dairy for a few days at a time but hadn't noticed a difference. Although the ultrasound didn't reveal any gallstones, I still thought that her recent attack might be related to her gallbladder, given its role in digesting fat and the amount of it she was eating, so I ordered a HIDA scan, a test that measures gallbladder function. Sure enough, the rate at which her gallbladder was releasing bile into the intestines—known as gallbladder ejection fraction—was exceedingly low, consistent with poor function. Despite two surgeons recommending she have her gallbladder removed, she didn't want to have surgery, and we were definitely on the same page there. We were both interested in how we could improve her gallbladder function rather than simply removing it.

We had a long discussion about her diet, and she realized she'd been snacking a lot more in the last year since her daughter had left for college and her business had gotten overwhelmingly busy. In the past she had made rice and beans or quinoa with vegetables for dinner most nights, but now it was often just cheese and crackers or yogurt, plus a couple of bags of chips and a few glasses of wine.

I recommended a drastic move: cut out dairy altogether for three months to see if we could improve her gallbladder function, which I felt sure was contributing to her pain and bloating. Since Carol was an accomplished cook with a great repertoire of vegetable dishes, she didn't need any help with menu planning or recipes, just gentle reminders that it didn't matter how successful her company was if she felt lousy, and that she really could leave work earlier so she'd have time to make dinner most nights.

My polite nagging was annoying but effective. After three months she was improved, but still not great. She had been diligent about avoiding dairy, not cheating even a little. The severe episodes of pain were gone, but she was still very bloated. I thought about other possibilities for what might be causing her bloating: she wasn't constipated; her thyroid function was good; and she didn't seem menopausal or even premenopausal, both of which can cause significant bloating. Endoscopy and colonoscopy were both normal, including biopsies for celiac disease and random biopsies throughout her GI tract looking for microscopic inflammation.

Carol asked whether a gluten-free diet (GFD) might help. A friend of hers had recently been diagnosed with celiac disease and was finally feeling well on a GFD after years of suffering. I told her it couldn't hurt and might help, so she had my blessing. The first four weeks she noticed no difference at all, except that life as a gluten-free vegetarian was challenging, especially when it came to snacks and eating out. I told her it might take a few months to see a difference, and with her friend's encouragement she decided to extend the experiment. At around week 6, her bloating virtually disappeared. She didn't have celiac disease, based on the negative blood test and normal biopsies of her small intestine done when she was still eating gluten, but her response to the GFD confirmed a diagnosis of gluten sensitivity.

Carol was gradually able to reintroduce some dairy into her diet, although she remained 100 percent gluten-free. Every now and again around the holidays she'd call to say her gallbladder was acting up, and I'd remind her to cut back on the dairy and cream sauces. She was still a little anxious about the possible need for gallbladder surgery, so we eventually repeated the scan. We found a well-functioning gallbladder with a high-normal ejection fraction.

These stories show some of the varied triggers and remedies for the cluster of symptoms we call IBS. With Mindy there was a potent intersection of psychology and physiology: stress was a major contributor, but it wasn't the whole story. Leslie's situation highlighted the importance of taking an honest and well-informed look at your diet, and how small additions like fruits, vegetables, and water can make a big difference. It also raised the uncomfortable issue of secondary gain through illness, something that can be subconscious and that both physicians and patients often struggle to address. There was less mind-body interplay with Carol, but the importance of steadfastness in searching for a diagnosis and dietary experimentation was major.

If I were to leave you with a final thought, it would be to recommend persistence, patience, and an open mind when it comes to investigating the factors that may be responsible for your IBS symptoms. My Gutbliss Plan is designed specifically with IBS in mind and offers a range of solutions that incorporate dietary strategies, lifestyle changes, and mind-body techniques. It's the ideal place to start if you're looking for innovative solutions in your quest for digestive wellness.

14

Could Your Gut Be Leaking?

WE'RE ALL ON A JOURNEY TRYING TO OPTIMIZE OUR HEALTH, BUT THERE can be differences in our destination and how we get there, depending on whom we travel with. There's still quite a philosophical divide between what conventional doctors consider real diagnoses and those that alternative practitioners tend to favor, and there's overdiagnosis of certain conditions on both sides.

Colon cancer, polyps, gallstones, hepatitis, and ulcers are diagnoses that have been around for a while. They cause changes in the GI tract that you can detect with an endoscope, ultrasound, or blood test—you can see and touch them. A diagnosis like leaky gut is much more nuanced; there's no specific test to diagnose it, and the evidence linking it to things that you can see or touch is murky. As a result, there's a lot of skepticism in the mainstream medical community about the legitimacy of leaky gut as a diagnosis, although, as evidence mounts that this is indeed a real and recognizable condition, opinions are slowly changing. In this chapter I'll tell you what's known about leaky gut, the syndrome that it causes, how it might be intimately connected to your bloating, and what you can do to try and remedy it.

Net Results: How Leaky Gut Happens

As I've described, the intestinal lining is like fishing net made of fine mesh with very small holes. Leaky gut, also known as increased intestinal permeability, refers to a condition where the holes in the net get bigger and allow more things to pass through that ordinarily couldn't. While one function of the intestines is nourishment—sending nutrients on their way to all the cells in your body—its other, equally important, function is protection: barring potentially harmful substances from circulating to the rest of your body.

When the holes in the intestinal net get larger, it compromises this barrier function, and bacteria, viruses, undigested food particles, and toxic waste products can leak through your intestinal lining into your bloodstream, where they may stimulate your immune system. In the absence of leaky gut, these substances normally wouldn't gain access to the rest of your body.

The immune system is a complicated network of cells and organs that protects the body from germs and other harmful substances. A crucial function of this network is the ability to distinguish between what's a normal part of your body and what's a foreign invader. Autoimmune disease develops when the body starts to react to its own tissue as though it were foreign. Genetic predisposition; dietary factors; exposure to viruses, bacterial infections, and environmental toxins; and loss of the intestinal barrier function are risk factors for developing autoimmune disease. As foreign substances leak through the intestinal membrane into the bloodstream, they are identified by the immune system as foreign. A cascade of events then ensues, resulting in inflammation in various parts of your body that can lead to a wide variety of symptoms, including bloating, cramps, fatigue, food sensitivities, flushing, achy joints, headache, and rashes.

In addition to stimulating an immune response, your body's receipt of nutrients may also be compromised. With leaky gut, poor absorption of nutrients often develops as a result of damage to the villi—the fingerlike projections in the small intestine responsible for absorbing nutrients—resulting in deficiencies and malnutrition even if you're eating a relatively healthy diet. Multiple food sensitivities are another hallmark of leaky gut,

Why Does Leaky Gut Happen?

Leaky gut, or increased intestinal permeability, is a condition that is still in its infancy in terms of what we know, but four factors—diet, chronic stress, inflammation, and bacterial imbalance—seem to play important roles. Some specifics:

- Eating a diet high in refined sugar, processed foods, preservatives, and chemicals has been associated with leaky gut. So has consumption of gluten, a protein found in wheat, rye, and barley.
- Excessive alcohol consumption can lead to damage of the intestinal lining.
- Chronic stress can lead to a weakened immune system, affecting your ability to fight off invading pathogens and worsening the symptoms of leaky gut.
- Medications such as aspirin and nonsteroidal anti-inflammatories (NSAIDs) that can damage the lining of your gut, antacids that change the pH, and steroids that alter the intestinal milieu, as well as antibiotics that kill off your essential good bacteria, are also associated with increased intestinal permeability.
- Dysbiosis, an imbalance between beneficial and harmful species in your gut that also includes overgrowth of yeast species, such as candida, and parasitic infection, is one of the leading theories explaining increased intestinal permeability (see Chapter 6, "Trouble in the Microbiome?").
- Radiation and chemotherapy can damage the lining of the intestine and are also risk factors for leaky gut.

as your immune system reacts to the incompletely digested particles of protein and fat that leak through the intestinal wall into the bloodstream. Having allergies to more than a dozen different foods should raise suspicion for leaky gut.

Increased intestinal permeability has also been described as a normal response to certain physiologic stressors, including intense exercise,

Gutbliss Solutions for Leaky Gut

There's no miracle cure for treating leaky gut, but there are things you can do if you think you're suffering from it that can help heal inflammation and restore the integrity of your gut lining. These solutions focus on *removing* offending agents, *replacing* good bacteria in the gut, and *repairing* the damaged intestinal lining.

Remove:

- My Gutbliss Plan incorporates an anti-inflammatory diet that eliminates refined sugars, dairy, gluten, alcohol, and artificial sweeteners—some of the biggest offenders when it comes to inflammation.
- Avoiding medications like NSAIDs, antibiotics, steroids, and other agents that can damage the intestinal lining is key.

Replace:

- Filling up on green leafy vegetables and other high-fiber foods that help to promote the growth of good bacteria is crucial. Fermented products like sauerkraut and kefir can also increase the ratio of good to bad bacteria.
- A regimen of robust probiotics like VSL#3 that contains large amounts of health-promoting *Bifidobacterium* and *Lactobacillus* species can help restore balance in the gut flora.

Repair:

- Consuming lots of anti-inflammatory essential omega-3 fatty acids in foods like fish, flax, hemp, wheat germ, and walnuts is a key part of an anti-inflammatory diet, since your body can't make them on its own. I recommend getting most of your nutrients from real food rather than supplements, but if allergies or the mercury content in fish is a concern, you can take 600 to 1,000 milligrams of a fish-oil supplement containing the omega-3 fatty acid docosahexaenoic acid (DHA). If you prefer not to eat animal products, you can substitute flax seed oil, chia seeds, and purslane, which contain the plant-based omega-3 alpha-linolenic acid (ALA) or take 600 to 1,000 milligrams of an ALA supplement.

- Glutamine is an amino acid that your cells use to make protein and as an energy source. Your intestinal lining cells are avid consumers of glutamine, which has been shown in some studies to help with intestinal injury after chemotherapy and radiation and may be beneficial in leaky gut. Safe doses in human studies range from 5 grams to about 15 grams daily.

Because we're still learning about leaky gut, these treatment recommendations are mostly drawn from anecdotal observation, and most aren't based on rigorous scientific studies. But they're sensible recommendations with a low risk of side effects that can lead to improvements in your overall health if you have increased intestinal permeability.

and we're still learning about what other factors contribute to the development of disease states in people with leaky gut. Increased intestinal permeability may potentially cause or worsen a number of other conditions, including celiac disease, inflammatory bowel disease (IBD, which includes Crohn's and ulcerative colitis), irritable bowel syndrome (IBS), rheumatoid arthritis, psoriasis, eczema, asthma, and perhaps even autism. Bloating also commonly occurs with leaky gut.

Leaky Gut Syndrome

Leaky gut syndrome is the presence of increased intestinal permeability, accompanied by symptoms, as a result of damage to the lining. It seems to be more common in the presence of dysbiosis and increased responsiveness of the immune system. A lot of the patients I see fall into this category. In addition to bloating and digestive distress, they frequently have other symptoms such as food allergies, chronic sinus infections and colds, achy joints, fatigue, or unexplained rashes. Typically they've been to multiple doctors, trying to make sense of their symptoms, and conventional tests and imaging studies have been unrevealing. There can be a feeling of hopelessness and despair, because the symptoms seem so disparate and unrelated. I'm also struck by how often there's a deep sense among people with these symptoms that they're slowly being poisoned.

Keep in mind that when food is inside your digestive tract, it's actually outside your body. The GI tract is a hollow tube, and substances have to be absorbed through the lining to gain access to your bloodstream, organs, and cells. Lots of things that find their way into your intestines are never meant to come into contact with the rest of your body, and under normal circumstances they're efficiently eliminated in your feces when you have a bowel movement. With leaky gut, they gain access to the inside of your body through the bloodstream, and all matter of mayhem may result.

Leaky gut is one of those diagnoses that bridge the gap between conventional and alternative medicine—it's in that as-yet-unmapped terrain between what we can see and touch and what we can feel in our bodies. My hunch is that as our knowledge grows, the theories behind leaky gut will become the foundation for lots of diseases that are widely prevalent in our society, in addition to bloating and GI distress.

15

Too Sweet for Your Own Good?

TEN MINUTES INTO MAUREEN'S FIRST VISIT WITH ME, I KNOW EXACTLY what's wrong. Not because I'm any smarter than the other three gastroenterologists she's seen, but because I've struggled with exactly the same problem. Maureen is an accomplished piano teacher and also runs a non-profit. She's an incredibly disciplined and industrious person who has three children and two jobs, and she also helps her husband with his business. Her middle child has serious medical problems, and she decided to pursue a more natural and holistic approach to his illness after the last pediatrician recommended long-term steroids. She believes in the concept of food as medicine, so there's very little junk food in their house. She buys organic produce and cooks a balanced dinner every night. Roast chicken with brown rice and steamed vegetables would be typical. The household has been soda-free for years; there are big bowls of fruit everywhere and not a bag of chips in sight.

Maureen's cheery demeanor turns sad as she describes her family history. Almost every relative was obese, diabetic, and died from cancer, including her parents, all their siblings, and her older sister, who struggled with her weight her entire life. Her sister weighed 270 pounds by age fifty, at which point she gave up battling her weight and ate whatever she wanted. She died two years later—at the same age Maureen is now.

Although Maureen isn't obese, she's definitely thirty or forty pounds overweight and terrified of her fate, given the family history. She also feels terrible—bloated and exhausted all the time. Fortunately, we're immediately on same page about nurture, rather than nature, being the overriding factor that determines our fate. She's not here to discuss her genetic bad luck. She's here to discuss how to change it.

Maureen says she's been steadily gaining weight at a rate of about five to ten pounds a year for the last several years and has no idea how to turn it around. "I feel like a fat-making machine," she tells me. She's seen lots of doctors who've told her the usual: she's stressed out and too busy; she's depressed; she needs to be more disciplined; she needs to make better choices; she needs to exercise more; she needs to control her portions. Weight Watchers helped her lose five pounds but she just couldn't seem to lose any more. She saw a naturopath who recommended lots of supplements, including one for her thyroid, which made her feel "weird," and none of the other herbs or vitamins helped her lose any weight. Blood tests have all been normal other than slightly elevated cholesterol and fasting blood glucose levels.

There's no question that Maureen's exercise and meal regimen are healthy. But Maureen has a secret: she is utterly and completely addicted to sugar. She wonders how it's possible for someone who's so incredibly disciplined in every other aspect of her life to have absolutely no control when it comes to this particular thing. She'll eat healthy meals throughout the day—then get out of bed at midnight and eat a huge bowl of ice cream. Or she'll eat a candy bar and cookies after dinner.

It's not so much that she binges—the amount of sugar she eats at one sitting isn't generally that excessive—it's the absolute compulsion she feels to have it every single day that's the problem. She can restrain herself for about twenty-four hours before the floodgates open and she literally *has* to have something sweet. In the last couple of years she hasn't been able to go more than forty-eight hours without dessert. Her nutritionally empty sugar calories are the main cause of her weight gain, and, as I'll explain, they're responsible for her bloating, too.

Chasing the Sugar Rush

Maureen's cravings are intense. The cycle goes something like this. She wakes up in the morning not thinking about sugar at all. She feels best when she eats a high-protein breakfast like eggs and smoked salmon, and she usually has a sandwich for lunch. Dinner is meat, chicken, or fish, a starch, a veg, and salad, followed by fruit. The cravings always come after dinner, like clockwork. No matter what she eats and how full she feels, she always wants dessert at night. And she always has it. She can usually resist until about ten p.m.; then she invariably breaks down and submits. Like many people who struggle with this kind of problem, her preference is to indulge late at night and by herself, usually watching television with the excuse of not being able to sleep.

Maureen feels high and elated even before she starts eating sugar. Just unwrapping the chocolate or thinking about the pint of ice cream in the freezer initiates feelings of intense pleasure. Once it's in front of her, she eats it pretty quickly, experiencing a giddy rush while enjoying every morsel, and sometimes going back for seconds. Within the hour comes the inevitable emotional response: remorse, guilt, and shame, followed by a steely resolve, telling herself this will surely be the last time she indulges like this. Twenty-four hours later, the cycle begins again.

Maureen has frequently set deadlines to quit her sugar habit—usually something auspicious, like her birthday or the New Year—but she's never been able to follow through. She's been watching herself get bigger and bigger and closer and closer to diabetes and the other problems she saw her parents and sister struggle with. She feels as if she's speeding toward some nightmarish destination without any ability to veer off course or slow down.

I know exactly how Maureen feels. I've run six marathons, survived medical school and residency, and endured sixteen hours of labor with a mostly ineffective epidural. All easy compared to not eating sugar. Lots and lots of sugar. There was a time when cookies, ice cream, and chocolate were the bane of my otherwise healthy existence. I'd have lentils, brown rice, and spinach for dinner, followed by a pint of Häagen-Dazs. Like Maureen, I wondered how it was possible for me to have such poor will-

The Not-So-Sweet Story

Most Americans consume close to their body weight in sugar per year. Sugars are carbohydrates made up of either one (monosaccharide), two (disaccharide), or multiple (oligosaccharide) linked molecules. Glucose and fructose, found primarily in fruits, vegetables, and industrial processed foods, and their slightly less sweet cousin, galactose, which is found primarily in dairy products and sugar beets, are simple monosaccharide sugars. Sucrose, also known as table sugar, is a disaccharide of glucose and fructose. Lactose is a disaccharide of glucose and galactose that occurs naturally in milk.

Sugar has been linked to obesity, diabetes, heart disease, dementia, tooth decay, and even some forms of cancer. Your sweet tooth may also be playing a major role in your bloating through a number of different mechanisms, including micronutrient deficiencies, inflammation, bacterial imbalance, and yeast overgrowth.

power when it came to sweets, as though my body was no longer under my control. What's important to understand is that when it comes to sugar, it's frequently not a matter of control but of addiction.

Maureen was imprisoned by her compulsion to have sugar, even though every rational part of her mind was telling her to try to resist. She felt sick and hungover after eating it, and she had a hunch it was responsible not just for her weight gain but also for her bloating and fatigue.

For anyone not convinced that this sort of addiction is real, read Neal Barnard, MD's book *Breaking the Food Seduction: The Hidden Reasons Behind Food Cravings—and 7 Steps to End Them Naturally*. Sugar releases natural opiates in your brain, which bind to receptors that activate the brain's pleasure center. The mechanism is almost identical to the effects of drugs like morphine and heroin, and not surprisingly, Maureen's behavior was in fact identical to someone addicted to morphine or heroin. She was hooked. The question was how to unhook her.

Kicking the Habit

The first thing I told her was that I didn't believe moderation was the answer to her sugar addiction. Just as I wouldn't tell an alcoholic that it's okay to have "just one" cocktail, or a cocaine addict that "a little" cocaine on the weekends was fine, so I wouldn't tell Maureen that she could have "a little" sugar—because for her, a little invariably led to a lot.

She was right about the sugar being responsible for a lot of her symptoms. The connection to her weight gain was obvious, but fluctuating blood sugar levels were also the main cause of her fatigue. High insulin levels confirmed with a blood test were consistent with the prediabetic state of insulin resistance and made me worry even more about diabetes and metabolic syndrome.

Because sugary foods often replace more nutritious ones and because sugar is devoid of the important nutrients your body needs to function well, overconsumption can lead to micronutrient deficiencies that have broad health implications. And diets high in sugar and other processed carbohydrates contribute to inflammation throughout the body and can suppress the immune system.

Maureen's sugar consumption was also a huge contributor to her bloating, as sugar is the preferred food for trillions of bacteria in your digestive tract. Too much of it sends them into a literal feeding frenzy, resulting in overgrowth of lots of undesirable species whose waste products include bloat-forming gas. As you learned in previous chapters, excessive sugar consumption can cause overgrowth of yeast species such as candida, which is associated with fatigue, leaky gut syndrome, and lots of other health problems.

Ironically, dysbiosis, an imbalance of gut bacteria that I suffered from during my sugar addiction, leads to intense cravings for more sugar (see Chapter 6, "Trouble in the Microbiome?"). Studies also show that changes in the bacterial composition of the gut associated with dysbiosis can make it substantially harder to lose weight and have even been implicated in depression.

Maureen was in trouble, or potentially so, on most of these counts. It was clear that whatever plan we embarked on was going to have to exclude sugar, at least in the short term.

Gutbliss Solutions for Sugar Addiction

I designed the same plan for Maureen that had worked for me and for many of my patients:

- Cut out the processed carbohydrates that cause a lot of insulin release: sugary foods such as cake, cookies, ice cream, and candy.
- Cut out starchy foods such as bagels, pasta, bread, white potato, and white rice, which are just glucose molecules, arranged differently.
- Keep healthy high-fiber carbs like beans, sweet potatoes, yams, brown rice, and quinoa.
- After-dinner fruit was a good idea, but we swapped out grapes, bananas, and clementines for more fibrous, less sweet choices like apples and pears, which wouldn't cause as high a spike in blood sugar. We could reintroduce a wider variety of fruit down the road, but for now it was important to get as much of the sugar as possible out of her system.

Lots of people turn to a low-carb lifestyle to help them lose weight as well as lose cravings. But it's easy to overdo the bacon, eggs, and hamburger patties, a route I definitely recommend avoiding if you're concerned about things like heart disease, cancer, and your overall health. I never recommend eliminating healthy carbohydrates. Instead:

- Incorporate lots of vegetables and "slow carbs" like legumes, sweet potatoes, and nuts.

Maureen was already a great vegetable eater and was used to cooking every day, which made what we were about to do much easier. This wasn't a complicated plan that required her to count carbohydrates, calories, or grams of fiber. In fact, there were no numbers at all—just certain foods that she needed to avoid, none of which were nutritionally beneficial anyway.

Once Maureen understood the connection between the high-sugar foods and her cravings and addiction, she was excited to begin. Her previous failures had nothing to do with self-control and everything to do with information; she had been trying to exercise portion control for a substance that was, for her, not controllable. I was optimistic about our new approach.

The first four days were brutal—she was essentially detoxing from sugar. She had terrible withdrawal symptoms consisting of severe cravings, hunger pangs, brain fog, exhaustion, and irritability. By day five, her withdrawal symptoms started to recede, and by the second week she was feeling much better. She'd been skeptical when I had initially told her that her sugar cravings could and would go away. But when she came for her follow-up visit three weeks later, she was a believer.

Maureen lost thirty pounds in four months and saw lots of other improvements in her health. Her blood sugar and cholesterol normalized, her bloating disappeared, and her energy level was much improved. But by far the most significant difference was her feeling of finally being in control over what she ate. She came to enjoy different kinds of endings to her meals: poached pears, nuts, or a bit of aged cheese.

After about six months Maureen spontaneously decided to test the waters with a slice of cake. The rush of sugar into her bloodstream within thirty minutes of eating it came as a shock. It was a sensation she had experienced daily in the past; in fact, she'd been a slave to this sugar high for years. But now it felt jarring and uncomfortable, and it reconfirmed that for her, avoiding sugar was the right path.

The point of Maureen's story is not to convince you that completely eliminating sugar is the key to good health, a trim waistline, and banishing your bloat. It's to share with you how for one particular person, identifying and eliminating a substance that was difficult to control and made her feel sick led to a lot of positive changes, both physically and emotionally. Plenty of healthy people eat dessert regularly or have a glass or two of wine with dinner every night and suffer no ill effects. From what I've seen, dependency and addiction aren't necessarily about how much of a substance you consume but about how much the substance consumes you.

I struggled to overcome my own sugar addiction, which caused terrible dysbiosis and cravings. In my case, the extra weight from empty sugar calories was ten pounds, not thirty, and I didn't have a compelling family history, high cholesterol, or prediabetes as Maureen did.

But I know unequivocally that when I cut out the sweet stuff, I feel my best. My skin is clearer and so is my brain; that yeasty itchy feeling goes away; I'm less bloated, more energetic, in a better mood; and I don't have a sugar hangover in the mornings.

But the most exhilarating change of all is liberation from the depressing cycle of cravings, indulgence, remorse, shame, and guilt.

Part of finding your gutbliss is examining those factors in your life—food and otherwise—that have a negative effect on how you feel. Identifying them and cutting back a little may be all you need. Or you may find that "none" is easier than "some." In that case, eliminating them altogether, as Maureen did, may be the right path for you.

16

Potholes on the GI Superhighway: Dealing with Diverticulosis

DIVERTICULOSIS IS ONE OF THE MOST COMMON DIGESTIVE CONDITIONS in people over fifty and a growing problem for younger people, too. If you have diverticulosis:

- You're probably bloated and having irregular bowel movements.
- You may have a feeling of incomplete evacuation after bowel movements.
- You may be alternating between too many bowel movements and too few, or having multiple unsatisfactory stools that leave you feeling constipated, despite lots of trips to the bathroom.
- Your gastroenterologist may have seen diverticulosis during your colonoscopy but still told you that your colon was "normal."
- You may have been diagnosed with irritable bowel syndrome (IBS), despite the presence of diverticulosis, leaving you scratching your head about what to do.

In this chapter I'll clear up any confusion about the significance of diverticulosis and go over the signs, symptoms, and potential complications. I'll also explain what causes diverticulosis to develop in the first place, why the condition is nonexistent in certain cultures, and how it can be prevented. Most important, if you're suffering from diverticulosis, I'll tell you what you need to know to unchain yourself from the bathroom, get rid of your bloating, and resurrect the days of effortless and bountiful bowel movements.

Lackluster Bowels

My patient Barbara is a fifty-seven-year-old judge who in the last several years has been very careful about her food: no trans fats, nothing processed, no red meat, organic fruits and vegetables from the farmer's market, and at least 20 grams of fiber a day. Given her healthy eating habits, she was completely perplexed as to why she was spending the better part of her day in the bathroom. Having a bowel movement had become a full-time job. The morning would get off to a reasonable start: a smallish log right after her morning tea, but things would deteriorate steadily after that with multiple, small, stuttering, pellet-sized poops that looked like rabbit droppings.

Each movement was accompanied by an annoying feeling of incomplete emptying. She could feel she had more stool inside, but she couldn't get it to come out. Invariably, within half an hour, it was back to the bathroom for more unsatisfying action.

Barbara was experiencing tenesmus, the medical term for incomplete evacuation that occurs when the colon can't fully rid itself of waste. And that's exactly how Barbara was feeling: toxic. She didn't want to go to the movies, she didn't want to go out to dinner, she didn't want to go to the gym, and she definitely wasn't in the mood when her husband got romantic. All she wanted was to get the stool out of her colon and into the toilet. She was bloated all the time, even after bowel movements, and was being driven to distraction by sitting on the toilet twenty times a day. Her erratic bathroom habits were interfering with her responsibilities in the courtroom, as she was constantly having to adjourn to take a bathroom break.

To add insult to injury, she was having a terrible time keeping her underwear clean because she was having problems with leakage she couldn't seem to control, as well as "wet gas." She had to wear a panty liner to catch stool stains and stray pellets and was going through mounds of toilet paper from endless wiping. She was fifty-seven, fit, and glamorous on the outside, but her insides felt old and lackluster—and the disparity was really starting to wear on her.

Things had been fine in the bathroom for Barbara until about two years ago, and they had been getting steadily worse since then. She thought her symptoms might have something to do with menopause, and she even worried about colon cancer based on how small and thin some of the stools were. She'd had her first screening colonoscopy five years ago when she was asymptomatic and had been told by the gastroenterologist who did the exam that everything was normal. Her internist concluded that she now had IBS and recommended that she consider stepping down from her position as a federally appointed judge to do something less stressful. But Barbara didn't feel stressed out by work. She felt stressed out by her bowel movements and rejected the notion that it was the other way around.

I asked Barbara to bring in all her old records for me to review, including the colonoscopy report from five years ago. It described a narrowed sigmoid colon due to bowel wall thickening and a few scattered, shallow diverticular orifices (i.e., potholes) in the lower part of the colon: classic early diverticulosis.

Diverticulosis: Widespread and Often Overlooked

More than a third of the population over age fifty in the United States has diverticulosis. Since that's the age when we recommend starting colonoscopy to screen for colon cancer, it's not surprising that it's one of the commonest things we see—often as an incidental finding in someone who's asymptomatic.

The good news is that diverticulosis isn't a risk factor for colon cancer, and it doesn't require medical intervention the way polyps, ulcerative colitis, or Crohn's do. The not-so-good news is that for this reason, it tends to get overlooked as an inconsequential finding, and it may not even get mentioned to someone who's asymptomatic, as was the case with Barbara after her first colonoscopy.

You yourself may have had a colonoscopy in which diverticulosis was seen but were told the colonoscopy was normal and that your symptoms were from IBS. I think part of the communication problem is that a colonoscopy is usually being done to look for colon cancer or polyps, so no cancer or polyps means a "normal exam." Or maybe if you had symptoms, you weren't vocal enough about them at the time of the colonoscopy, leading your gastroenterologist to discount them and not put two and two together.

In addition, some doctors see diverticulosis as a natural part of the aging process of the colon—like wrinkles or gray hair—nothing that requires a great deal of discussion. Others just aren't well versed on the kinds of symptoms diverticulosis can cause, focusing instead on more dramatic complications like diverticulitis—infected or inflamed diverticular pockets. This is why I'm always interested in seeing the actual report when someone's had a previous colonoscopy: "normal" doesn't always mean nothing's wrong.

I decided to repeat Barbara's colonoscopy because it had been five years since her last one and her symptoms were quite severe. When I took a look at her colon, the diverticulosis was still there (it doesn't go away, but we can prevent progression and complications), but it was much more extensive than on her previous exam. Instead of the little dimples of five years ago, she now had large craterlike potholes, giving the lower half of her colon a Swiss cheese appearance.

It turned out that Barbara's mother, aunt, and paternal grandfather all had diverticulosis. While diverticulosis isn't genetic, it's extremely common in the developed world based on our diet, and people from the same family tend to eat the same way, so they have the same risk factors for developing it.

Causes

Diverticulosis is a result of a diet that's too low in fiber and too high in animal products. High pressure develops in the wall of the colon when it has to contract more vigorously to expel small, hard stool characteristic of a low-fiber diet. This leads to small bulges, which eventually become the orifices of diverticulosis, frequently referred to as pouches, pockets, or

The Diet Debate

The role of diet is often downplayed in Western medicine, while the role of pharmaceutical intervention is emphasized. Some studies have tried to dispel the notion that colon cancer and diverticulosis are associated with a low-fiber, high-animal-fat diet, despite the fact that population-based studies clearly confirm them as risk factors. Most of these studies use voluntary recall from patients who claim to be eating a high-fiber diet and nonetheless have diverticulosis, as proof that the fiber connection isn't valid. But just as we tend to overestimate how much we're exercising when asked, so we tend to overestimate how much fruits, vegetables, and other healthy foods we're consuming and underestimate the amount of meat, fatty foods, and desserts, especially in the context of completing a medical questionnaire. So it's not surprising that some of these studies suggest that diverticulosis is common even in the setting of a high-fiber diet.

potholes. Thickening of the muscular wall of the colon, especially the sigmoid, also occurs from all the vigorous contractions to try to expel this small, hard stool.

In sub-Saharan Africa and other parts of the world where people can't afford animal products and eat a diet high in unprocessed fiber with lots of root vegetables and legumes, they have large bulky stools two or three times a day and very low rates of diverticulosis and colon cancer. These impressive stools drop effortlessly from the rectum, requiring no vigorous contractions and leaving no messy residue requiring reams of toilet paper, a phenomenon I refer to as *the clean wipe*. In the United States we recommend eating between 25 and 35 grams of fiber a day, but if you're eating anything resembling the Standard American Diet (SAD), you're only getting about 10 grams and you're probably suffering from smeary stools and messy cleanup. You're also at risk for developing digestive problems like diverticulosis and colon cancer.

There's also the issue of what people ate in childhood, which, in Barbara's case, was very different from what she was eating now. She grew up in the Midwest eating a meat-and-potatoes diet—greens were garnish to put around the roast beef. The foundation for diverticulosis is laid down way before the symptoms finally appear. I'm seeing more and more patients in their twenties and thirties with diverticulosis, a disease that's supposed to strike late in middle age. I take it as a worrisome sign that what we're eating in America is not only failing to nourish us but is also making us sick.

How the Damage Happens

So we know what causes diverticulosis, but how exactly does the diverticulosis cause bloating and bowel problems? Diverticulosis can occur anywhere along the length of the colon, but it's most common in the sigmoid, the part of the colon that works the hardest to push formed stool into the rectum. All that pushing causes the sigmoid to become thickened, as well as full of potholes. Stool can get stuck in these potholes, sometimes for days or even weeks at a time. The combination of potholes filled with stool and a narrow, thickened colon makes you feel really full, bloated, and uncomfortable. The sigmoid is located in the lower left part of the abdomen and sometimes extends across the midline to just above the pelvic bone, and that's where most people have discomfort. On exam I can usually feel a thick sigmoid colon, full of stool.

So now your thick sigmoid colon full of stool is pressing down on your rectum and creating the strong sensation that you have to have a bowel movement. But there isn't enough stool actually in the rectum to trigger contraction of the muscles necessary for defecation to happen. So you're in and out of the bathroom because you have all this pressure from the sigmoid colon but not enough stool in the rectum. It feels like you have to go, but very little is actually coming out of your half-empty rectum. Finally the potholes begin to empty, and you start to have a little action, but it takes multiple trips because the potholes don't all empty at once. If you're lucky, you may be able to squeeze out a pellet here and there or thin toothpaste-like ribbons of stool, but most of the time things are pretty unsatisfactory.

Having multiple small bowel movements but still feeling constipated is the most annoying symptom of diverticulosis and also the most characteristic. Bowel movements after meals and in the evening are especially

Diverticulitis: A Complication of Diverticulosis

Diverticulitis refers to infection or inflammation of the potholes. The longer the stool sits in the pockets, the greater the risk for infection developing, so constipation is definitely to be avoided, as are nonsteroidal anti-inflammatory drugs (NSAIDs), which increase the risk of both bleeding and infection. These bouts can be treated in a number of ways: bowel rest, a liquid diet, antibiotics (if severe pain, fever, or an elevated white blood cell count are present), and analgesia. Worst-case scenarios include surgery to remove an affected area.

annoying. Eating stimulates contraction and as the day progresses, the products of digestion move through your colon, filling your already-full sigmoid and stimulating it to contract—not comfortable at all.

People are usually quite puzzled by this situation and wonder whether they have a parasite or some sort of blockage because they can feel the stool up there, even though it doesn't seem to want to come out. The longer stool sits in the potholes, the more it's fermented by bacteria, producing lots of hydrogen and methane gas that make an already full and thickened colon feel even more bloated and uncomfortable. When the stool finally makes its exit, the first part can be hard from all the water that's been reabsorbed from it while it's been waiting to come out, but the subsequent stool is often soft from all the fermentation and may fall apart in the toilet.

Because the sigmoid can be very long and twisty, it sits low and deep, falling into the pelvis and even crossing over to the right side. That's why symptomatic diverticulosis can sometimes feel like a bladder or ovarian problem. In fact, a thickened sigmoid colon can press against the bladder, irritating it and leading to frequent urination and a feeling of pressure. Barbara had been told she had interstitial cystitis and was treated with antibiotics multiple times for nonexistent urinary tract infections. Complications also include bleeding from the rupture of superficial blood vessels inside the potholes.

Treating Diverticulosis

Fortunately, if you're in the early phases of diverticulosis, dietary improvement—an undoing of the low-fiber, nutrient-poor diet that may have led to this problem in the first place—can have incredible results. Barbara had so far been spared bleeding or infectious complications from her diverticulosis, but she was still very symptomatic just from the presence of the potholes. So when she and I sat down to formulate a plan to get her out of the bathroom, one of the things I asked her to do was aim for more than 30 grams of fiber, not counting any of the grams of fiber from cereal, pasta, baked goods, or bread.

Not all fiber is created equal when it comes to laxation, a fancy term for moving the bowels. Unprocessed, naturally occurring foods like fruits, vegetables, squash, yams, nuts, seeds, and beans provide us with the type of fiber that has much more bang for the buck than what we get from processed sources like breakfast cereals, whole wheat bread, fiber bars, chips, and baked goods, no matter what the nutritional label on the package says.

Even though Barbara was eating a fair amount of fruits and vegetables, a lot of it was tropical fruits, such as pineapple and bananas, and salad with iceberg lettuce. These foods have valuable nutrients but not that much fiber. I recommended adding apples, pears, and berries and tossing spinach, chickpeas, and raw veggies into her salads. But she still needed some help getting to 30 grams. I'm not keen on processed forms of fiber from cereal or baked goods or food manufacturers' practice of adding it to things like yogurt or candy bars where it doesn't naturally occur and has questionable benefits, but I am a huge fan of fiber supplements. A daily tablespoon or two of ground psyllium husk can make straining and incomplete evacuation things of the past. The wonderful thing about fiber is that as you start to consume more of it, not only do you start having bigger stools that pass out more easily, but your risk for developing serious conditions such as heart disease, cancer, stroke, and diabetes also decreases.

I started Barbara on a tablespoon of ground psyllium in the morning and after a week added a second dose at night. I warned her that things might get worse before they got better, which they did. The first two

Gutbliss Solutions for Diverticulosis

If your symptoms sound like diverticulosis:

First of all, find out if you really have it. If you've had a colonoscopy or a CAT (computerized axial tomography) scan, ask if it showed diverticulosis or thickening in the sigmoid colon, which could be an early sign. If you haven't had any testing, ask your doctor whether he or she thinks you should have a colonoscopy to investigate your symptoms.

Fortunately, complications from diverticulosis like diverticulitis and bleeding are the exception rather than the norm, and most people will never require hospitalization, antibiotics, or surgery for this condition. The most helpful tactics for getting the symptoms under control are still the basics:

A high-fiber diet aiming for 30 grams of fiber from natural sources like fruits, vegetables, legumes, nuts, seeds, and unprocessed whole grains. See my 10-Day Gutbliss Plan (Chapter 23) for specifics on how to accomplish this.

Try my "recipe" for adding psyllium husk to your diet:

- 1 teaspoon of finely ground psyllium once a day in the morning, mixed with at least 8 ounces of liquid and followed by an additional 8-ounce glass of water

You may feel full and even more bloated the first few days, but after a week your body should be used to the increased fiber. Then:

- After a week, add a second teaspoon in the middle of the day.
- After two weeks, add a third teaspoon at bedtime.
- Be sure to follow each dose with an additional glass of water.
- Plenty of water to keep the stool soft—at least a liter a day.
- Exercise to encourage peristaltic movement through the colon.
- Eliminating gluten and dairy can also be helpful strategies and have led to improved bowel habits in many of my patients.

weeks, as her body adjusted to the added amount of fiber, she was more bloated and constipated than she'd ever been and on the verge of firing me as her gastroenterologist. But then something remarkable happened.

Her bowel movements started to get bigger. Much bigger. Fill-the-toilet-bowl bigger. Clog-the-toilet-bowl bigger on one occasion. And they also started to get less frequent. Twenty trips became ten. And ten became five. And five settled into three really good stools.

Even though Barbara still had a feeling of fullness from her thickened sigmoid colon, she was much less bloated, not spending all day in the bathroom, and having three stools instead of twenty, and she was pretty happy with that.

Stool nirvana is different for everyone. By being mindful of initial signs and symptoms and making a habit of eating in the way we discuss in this book, you'll have the edge on preventing diverticulosis, catching it early, or stopping it in its tracks.

17

Of All the Gall: Bloating and Your Gallbladder

ROSE WAS IN A BIG HURRY WHEN SHE CAME TO SEE ME. GALLBLADDER surgery was looming on the horizon and she needed answers fast. As I read through her initial food journal that I have new patients fill out, I tried to maintain a neutral expression.

She had been having a cheese Danish with a latte for breakfast, a turkey and provolone sandwich for lunch, and steak, chicken, or cheese pasta for dinner, with ice cream for dessert. Occasionally she'd have an apple for a snack, but usually it was a chocolate bar, cookies, or frozen yogurt. By way of explanation, she told me that her husband didn't like vegetables and her daughter was a picky eater, so they invariably ended up eating a lot of high-fat foods that appealed to everyone.

I've seen lots of food journals in my time (and mine certainly isn't always pristine), but Rose's was Exhibit A for what not to eat if you're bloated and have a sick gallbladder. I say "sick" and surgeons say "diseased" because they're usually interested in making a case for removing it, and I'm usually interested in making a case for improving it. Rose was bloated, frustrated, and in pain, and she had just been told that she needed to have her gallbladder removed ASAP.

Medical textbooks and Web sites often refer to the gallbladder as a

The "Leave It In/Take It Out" Debate

The year 1997 was one of big change in the surgical world. For decades gallbladders had been removed by making a large diagonal abdominal incision, requiring a three- to six-day hospital stay plus six weeks of recovery at home. All that changed with the advent of laparoscopic cholecystectomy. With a few tiny punctures, surgical instruments and a camera could be inserted into the abdominal cavity and the gallbladder pulled out through a small hole. Hospital stay was reduced to twenty-four hours, with only a week of additional recovery. The surgery itself took less time, with decreased infection rates, faster healing, and less scar tissue.

But these advances would ultimately lead to changes that weren't necessarily beneficial for all patients. Since the laparoscopic technique was introduced, the number of cholecystectomies performed in the United States has increased by almost 50 percent. Is it an incredible coincidence that just as the surgery got easier, so many more people developed gallbladder problems—or are there additional reasons to explain why people are losing their gallbladders in record numbers?

Philosophically, some surgeons believe an ounce of prevention is worth a pound of cure and therefore have a low threshold for gallbladder removal. Then there's the unsavory issue of profit. It's comforting for us as consumers of health care to think that our providers are always acting in our best interest, and most of the time I think they are, but, unfortunately, that's not always the case. Technological advances in medicine always generate excitement, and doctors don't always follow guidelines designed to prevent unnecessary procedures. So if you aren't asking lots of questions and considering alternate options, you might find yourself facing a procedure that may be nifty but not necessary.

nonessential organ. Nothing could be farther from the truth. Can you live without your gallbladder? Absolutely, but there's a good chance your digestion will never be the same, and you'll be even more bloated than you were before. There's no question that gallbladders can be problematic— from causing annoying but relatively manageable troubles like gas and bloating to life-threatening situations like gangrenous cholecystitis. It can be tricky deciding whether you're better off with yours in or out. In this chapter I'll go over what makes your gallbladder sick and how to nurse it back to health (it's simpler than you think), as well as the pros and cons of holding on to it when it's literally being a pain.

Master Fat Blaster

So what does the gallbladder do anyway, and if almost a million people in the United States alone have theirs removed each year, how vital an organ can it be?

Every piece of tissue in your body is there for a reason. In the case of the digestive tract, each organ plays a unique role in the complex process of digestion. Even the appendix, which many regard as a vestigial organ that has outlived its usefulness, is now known to be an important site for storage of beneficial gut bacteria and a source of immune tissue. The gallbladder is located under the rib cage on the right side of the abdomen, just below the liver. It's a small sac about the size and shape of a pear, and its main job is to store and release bile, which is made in the liver.

When you eat, food gets churned up in the stomach into small particles called chyme, which travels into the duodenum, the first part of the small intestine. In response to the chyme, receptors in the duodenum secrete the hormone cholecystokinin, which stimulates the gallbladder to contract and release bile. Bile helps with the absorption of fat in the chyme by emulsifying it—basically mixing the fat with the watery secretions of the intestines, much like dishwashing liquid helps dissolve grease on plates.

Like most of our organs, gallbladder function is based on feedback loops. A high-fat meal causes more bile release and a low-fat meal causes less. It's straightforward and works well when you eat a reasonable diet and avoid too much saturated fat and other cholesterol-laden foods. What's too much? Rose's Exhibit A diet: a cheese Danish with a latte for breakfast, turkey and provolone for lunch, and steak, chicken, or cheese pasta for dinner. Plus ice cream for dessert.

Cholesterol is present only in animal products, and if there's too much in your diet, it crystallizes in the bile, causing gallstones. Most of us don't need to follow complicated guidelines about how many grams of saturated versus unsaturated fat to eat—our bodies give us all the feedback we need: when things start to go wrong with our gallbladder, it's usually a sure sign that we need to make some changes.

Cholesterol Made Simple

The food industry has gone to great lengths to set up complex hierarchies of good, better, and best when it comes to cholesterol, with fish at the top of most people's pyramids and red meat at the bottom. But the truth is, there's not a huge difference between beef, chicken, or fish when it comes to cholesterol.

A small serving (about four ounces) of

- lean ground beef has 78 milligrams of cholesterol
- beef sirloin has 89 milligrams of cholesterol
- white meat skinless chicken has 85 milligrams of cholesterol
- a pork chop has 85 milligrams of cholesterol
- salmon has 63 milligrams of cholesterol

Of course, if you're eating wild fish, there are additional benefits, such as omega-3 fatty acids, which have anti-inflammatory properties. But the idea that one kind of flesh is significantly better for us than another is a construct that leaves us scrambling for chicken breast over hamburger when we really should be thinking about plants versus animals. For most of us, simply increasing the amount of plants in our diet, especially the green leafy kind, and cutting back on animal products will take care of whatever gallbladder issues we have, give us enviable cholesterol levels, and help prevent a host of other problems, including heart disease and cancer.

The Academy of Nutrition and Dietetics (formerly the American Dietetic Association) recommends that we consume less than 300 milligrams of cholesterol daily. The difference between an 85-milligram chicken breast and an 89-milligram piece of sirloin pales in comparison to the fact that fruits, vegetables, nuts, seeds, beans, yams, potatoes, rice, and grains have *zero* cholesterol. It makes the math a lot simpler.

What Can Go Wrong with Gallbladders

Gallbladder problems can be divided into three main categories:

1. acute gallbladder infection or inflammation (acute cholecystitis),
2. chronic gallbladder dysfunction (cholecystopathy), or
3. gallstones.

To make things a little more complicated, gallstones can be present or absent with either of the first two conditions, as can something called sludge, which is thicker than bile but not as thick as gallstones. Also, gallstones aren't caused by cholesterol only; bilirubin and calcium can form pigment stones and are common in conditions like sickle-cell anemia.

When gallstones slip into the bile ducts, they can cause a blockage and disrupt the flow of bile. Depending on where they end up, they can also block the ducts that drain the liver and pancreas, causing jaundice and pancreatitis. If the flow of bile from the gallbladder is obstructed, it can become swollen and tender, like a big pus-filled pimple—a condition called cholecystitis. Fever, severe pain, or unstable vital signs raise the concern that your gallbladder may burst open, and surgery to avoid that possibility is usually the best option for acute cholecystitis.

If a gallstone is blocking your bile duct but you're not as acutely ill, it may pass through on its own, or you may need a procedure called an ERCP (endoscopic retrograde cholangiopancreatography) where the gallbladder is left in place but the bile ducts are swept clean with small pipe cleaner–like wires. Removal of the gallbladder down the road may be recommended for recurrent obstructing gallstones.

"SILENT" VERSUS HARMFUL GALLSTONES

Now here's what you really need to know about gallstones: if I lined one hundred random people up against a wall and did an ultrasound on them—the simplest and least invasive way to detect gallstones—between ten and fifteen of them would have a positive test. Of that 10 to 15 percent of the population with gallstones, the vast majority will have no symptoms whatsoever that are attributable to their gallstones. They may have nonspecific digestive symptoms, as many of us do from time to time, like bloating, nausea, or mild abdominal discomfort, but 75 to 80 percent of people with gallstones have no symptoms that are a direct result of the gallstones.

If you're one of those people with "silent" gallstones, your risk of having an acute gallbladder attack is only about 1 percent. All too often these nonspecific digestive symptoms are wrongly attributed to the gallbladder, which is innocently going about doing its job, not posing a threat to anybody. When the gallbladder is removed in that setting, the symptoms that were never caused by the gallbladder in the first place are clearly still going to be there after surgery.

But what if your symptoms are caused by your gallbladder, and you're having them after every meal? In the absence of a condition indicating a clear need for surgery, such as acute cholecystitis, gallstones that keep obstructing the ducts, or severe symptoms from a poorly functioning gallbladder, I still say at least *try* to hold on to your gallbladder. Here's why: symptoms like bloating, abdominal discomfort, and nausea may not be resolved by simply taking out the gallbladder, because even when it's functioning poorly and causing those symptoms, removing it doesn't address the fundamental problem behind why it's not working.

Remember, the gallbladder doesn't make bile; it just stores it for the liver. If the problem is abnormal bile production, then the factors contributing to that need to be addressed. In addition to too much or poor-quality fats, other causes include overconsumption of carbohydrates leading to imbalanced carbohydrate and lipid metabolism, rapid weight loss, diabetes, alcohol, birth control pills, or hormone replacement therapy (see "Risk Factors for Gallstones" on page 168). These factors may ultimately affect your gallbladder, but they're really problems that affect the body as a whole. Removing the gallbladder without remediating them doesn't solve the problem, as demonstrated by the fact that up to 20 percent of people have recurrence of symptoms after their gallbladder is removed.

When Your Gallbladder Is an Innocent Bystander

Unfortunately, a lot of people find out after surgery that their gallbladder wasn't the cause of their bloating. Conditions such as bacterial over-

Risk Factors for Gallstones

- Age
- Alcohol
- Bile duct strictures
- Birth control pills
- Cholangitis (brown pigment bile duct stones)
- Cirrhosis
- Crohn's disease
- Diabetes
- Diet: high fat/low fiber/high carbohydrate
- Ethnicity (Pima Indians)
- Female gender
- Genetics (gene mutation)
- History of abdominal surgery
- Hormone replacement therapy
- Ileal resection (black pigment stones)
- Infections (*Helicobacter* species, malaria)
- Medications (calcineurin inhibitors, cholesterol-lowering drugs, octreotide, ceftriaxone)
- Metabolic syndrome
- Obesity
- Organ transplantation
- Physical inactivity
- Pregnancy
- Rapid weight loss/surgery for obesity
- Sickle-cell anemia
- Spinal cord injury
- Total parenteral nutrition (intravenous nutritional therapy)
- Vitamin B_{12}/folic acid deficient diet (black pigment stones)

growth, acid reflux, *H. pylori* infection, stomach ulcers, gluten sensitivity, lactose intolerance, delayed stomach emptying, and parasites can mimic the signs and symptoms of a poorly functioning gallbladder, causing nausea, bloating, and abdominal pain. By far the biggest problem I see after surgery is the continued presence of the original symptoms, reported in some studies in almost half of all patients who have their gallbladder removed. Even worse, in addition to the original symptoms, which might have been mistakenly attributed to the gallbladder, new symptoms may develop when the main organ responsible for bile secretion and fat absorption is gone. Without the gallbladder to store and secrete just the right amount of bile after meals, there's either too much or not enough bile being circulated. Severe bloating and diarrhea after eating is what most of my patients complain of, but some people also report constipation or nausea. If you thought you had problems with fatty meals before your gall-bladder was removed, you may have even more difficulty after. Granted, my patient population is a bit skewed. People who have their gallbladder removed for an appropriate indication, get relief, and feel fine don't have any reason to come see me. I see their counterparts: people who didn't get relief and may be feeling even worse.

What About Elective Gallbladder Surgery?

Most of the rise in gallbladder surgery has been in people with what we call "soft indications," that is, a suboptimally functioning gallbladder or asymptomatic gallstones rather than an acutely infected gallbladder or severe dysfunction. A study of fifty-four thousand gallbladder surgeries in Pennsylvania found that the number of procedures done in patients with minimal or no symptoms had increased by more than 50 percent since the advent of laparoscopic surgery. But is preventing severe attacks before they occur a good idea? Well-meaning doctors might show you ultrasound pictures of stones in your gallbladder. They might tell you a story or two of a patient who died from massive infection because a gallstone slipped out of the gallbladder into their bile duct and caused a blockage. But the fascinating statistic, published in the *New England Journal of Medicine* (*NEJM*), is that waiting and having emergency surgery if your bile duct becomes blocked is actually safer than proceeding with elective surgery to prevent a blocked duct in the future. More people die from elective gallbladder surgery than from emergency surgery. This turns prevailing wisdom on its head, since most of us assume that elective surgery is safer than emergency surgery and therefore might choose the former to prevent the latter.

The study also underscores the best medical advice I can give you: if it ain't broke, consider not fixing it. Well-informed observation—that is, you and your doctor paying close attention to any change in your symptoms—is sometimes a great idea, and as the *NEJM* article illustrated, having surgery now for something that could go wrong in the future may not be the best decision. As a physician, the idea of removing parts of your body in the absence of a really compelling indication, such as cancer or intractable disease, strikes me as pretty drastic. We've seen examples throughout history of tonsils, uteruses, and thyroid glands being preemptively removed with good intentions. The results are almost always the same: a decline in your health that no amount of antibiotics, estrogen supplements, or thyroid medication can improve. Our focus should be on figuring out where things went wrong and why, and fixing the underlying problem, instead of just removing the organ and hoping for the best. You need your organs. Try to hold on to them as long as possible and then, ideally, pass them on to someone else when you're passing on and no longer need them. Elective surgery for silent gallstones isn't usually necessary, and it's almost never a good idea.

The Magic of Change

As Rose began making these changes, our office visits were all about food, stress, and balance. She fell off the wagon a bunch of times, but when her symptoms returned, rather than getting down on herself for "failing," they reminded her of how far she'd come in taking steps to feel so much better. Her gallbladder attacks became less frequent and less intense.

Still, it was a little unbelievable to her, this direct association between what she was eating and how she was feeling. It felt like some sort of magic trick. About six months into the dietary changes, however, when we repeated the HIDA scan, it showed that her gallbladder ejection fraction was now well within the normal range. The magic was working!

Rose's household remained somewhat divided in terms of her more plant-based diet versus her husband's high-fat animal protein consumption. Over time they agreed to disagree and made their peace with the fact that they had different philosophical beliefs when it came to food as medicine. But the proof was in the pudding as Rose and her gallbladder continued to function well.

If you think your gallbladder may not be working quite right, by all means see a doctor and get an ultrasound, HIDA scan, or any other tests or blood work he or she might recommend. If your problems are more pressing—fever, severe pain, tenderness, abnormal lab values—and you're told that your gallbladder needs to come out, that's probably sage advice. But if you're one of the millions of people with symptoms like bloating, feeling full after meals, mild nausea, and abdominal discomfort, consider the possibility that your gallbladder itself may not be the culprit, even if you have gallstones, and that the problem may be elsewhere. And even when it seems like your gallbladder *is* the problem, make sure it's not an innocent bystander, caught up in a tangled web of other problems, such as too much consumption of high-fat foods and not enough physical activity. Changing what you eat and how you live is hard, but just do what Rose did and take things one bite at a time. It's so worth it, particularly when it allows you to hold on to your organs.

Gutbliss Solutions for Gallbladder Issues

As it turned out, Rose didn't have gallstones; she had a poorly functioning gallbladder with a low ejection fraction on HIDA scan, which meant it wasn't releasing bile very efficiently. I've seen lots of people in similar situations that with dietary modification not only improve their symptoms but dramatically improve their HIDA scan ejection fraction, too.

Bite by Bite: One Fruit/One Veg a Day

So we did what we always do with people who are trying to make big scary changes in their diet and, ultimately, in their lives. We took it bite by bite. We started with the concept of one fruit/one vegetable a day that had worked well for so many of my patients. Not only are these foods cholesterol-free, but some of them can actually help to lower cholesterol. Plant sterols block the absorption of cholesterol in the body, and studies show that vegetarians and people who follow a plant-based diet have much lower cholesterol levels. If you have high cholesterol, I'm not suggesting that you stop taking your medication without checking with your doctor. But I am suggesting that shifting to a plant-based diet may not only help lower your cholesterol but also reduce the likelihood of developing gallbladder disease.

Trim the Fat

We also agreed that Rose would eliminate the one item that was really a problem: her beloved dairy that she was overdosing on. Dairy is quick, convenient, and delicious. It's so easy to grab some cheese and crackers or a Greek yogurt, drink a latte or cappuccino, or sprinkle some shaved Parmesan or feta in your salad. But the amount of dairy you're consuming can really start to add up, and the GI tract may have a hard time digesting it. Dairy is the biggest contributor to fat in the American diet, which is why even vegetarians who eat a lot of it aren't immune from developing gallbladder problems.

Rose wasn't sure she'd be able to follow through 100 percent with the plan, but she agreed to try. Within a few weeks, her breakfast cheese Danish had become a bowl of steel-cut oatmeal. She prepared one big pot on a Monday morning and it lasted her until Friday, reheating portions on the stove with a little almond milk. Some days she added berries, other days nuts and seeds or bananas. Lunchtime turkey and cheese morphed into butternut squash or lentil soup that she made in large batches and froze in single serving-size portions she could thaw and heat at home or at work. Dinner was still meat, chicken, or fish, but now it was always accompanied by cooked green veggies and sweet potatoes or squash.

Get Moving

Instead of driving, Rose started commuting to work by metro, which involved a lot more walking. A European study published in 2010 revealed that people with gallstones who were physically active had fewer symptoms than their sedentary counterparts, and the overall risk reduction for gallbladder problems was as much as 70 percent in the most active group. These beneficial effects seem to be synergistic with nutritional modifications like a high-fiber, low-fat diet. Studies also show that exercise can both prevent gallstones from forming and reduce symptoms if you already have them.

Seriously Bloated

HOW DO YOU KNOW IF YOUR BLOATING ISN'T JUST A NUISANCE BUT A sign of something more worrisome? In this chapter, the term *seriously bloated* doesn't refer to the severity of your symptoms but to the underlying cause: you're seriously bloated when your symptoms are caused by a condition that requires immediate medical attention. The symptoms that accompany serious bloating aren't necessarily worrisome on their own, but certain combinations of symptoms, in the right setting, particularly if you have a compelling family history or additional risk factors, may point to a more serious diagnosis that needs further investigation. In this chapter I'll discuss the warning signs and symptoms that might indicate something ominous, and the ten diagnoses that you need to know about if you're concerned that you might be seriously bloated.

There's no question that we're talking about serious subjects here. Fortunately, even aggressive cancers and other major illnesses, when caught early enough, can be treated and often cured. If you have any concerns at all about whether your bloating may represent something more than just a bothersome symptom, don't hesitate to seek immediate medical attention.

Warning Signs

WEIGHT LOSS

Weight loss is one of the main warning signs for serious bloating. If you find yourself losing more than a few pounds without changing your diet or starting a new exercise regimen, that should be a cause for concern, especially if it's 10 percent or more of your body weight. Weight loss can be a result of a tumor or scar tissue that's pressing on the intestines, making you full after just a small amount of food, or it can be from substances secreted by a cancer somewhere in your body that suppresses your appetite.

WEIGHT GAIN

A large tumor in the abdomen or pelvis can cause significant weight gain and be a sign of serious bloating. Other types of tumors, such as those in the pituitary gland in the brain, can lead to weight gain because of improper hormone regulation. Chronic inflammation in the body can lead to weight gain because of elevated levels of cortisol, the stress hormone.

ASCITES

Ascites is an abnormal buildup of fluid in the abdomen or pelvis, and it can cause weight gain and a rapidly expanding waistline. Ascites is usually caused by liver disease, but about 10 percent of the time cancer is the culprit and the ascites is malignant. A large amount of ascites may make you look and feel like you're several months pregnant. How can you tell if your bloat is from air or ascites? When you lie flat on your back, ascites fluid will fall to the sides and accumulate in your flanks, whereas air will rise to the top of your belly. If you think you may have ascites, you should seek immediate medical attention because, although the causes of ascites are not all cancerous, they're all serious. The combination of bloating and jaundice, which turns the eyes and skin yellow, should raise suspicions for cancer that has spread to the liver, although it can also occur with benign forms of liver disease.

PAIN

Pain is obviously a subjective sensation, but you know your body the best, so you're the most qualified to decide whether your pain is significant. You may not know what the diagnosis is, but trust your instincts if you're having abdominal or pelvic pain with your bloating that feels different from the occasional discomfort you might get from eating too much or from your period. If the first doctor doesn't take you seriously, try a second, third, and fourth. Keep going until you get a proper evaluation and reassurance that all is well.

BOWEL OBSTRUCTION

Severe abdominal pain and bloating that occur suddenly, especially if accompanied by nausea and vomiting, may be due to a bowel obstruction from scar issue or from a tumor pressing on the bowel. Obstructions require immediate medical attention to avoid complications, such as bowel perforation, which can be fatal. A bowel obstruction down in the colon will cause pain, but an obstruction higher up at the level of the stomach or small intestine may also cause vomiting as the bowel tries to empty its contents. Obstructions are painful because the bowel above the blocked area stretches as it fills with food and digestive juices. The pain is usually intense and may occur in waves as full, distended loops of bowel try to push their contents through the obstructed area. Sometimes an obstruction develops more slowly and doesn't completely block the passage of stool and air, in which case the pain may not be as severe and may develop over time, but will still be associated with significant bloating, discomfort, and often a feeling of fullness.

BLEEDING

Blood in your stool, vaginal bleeding in between periods, or postmenopausal vaginal bleeding can all be associated with serious bloating. The most common causes for these symptoms (hemorrhoids, an irregular menstrual cycle, or benign conditions such as endometriosis) aren't always the most serious, but bleeding should always be evaluated because it can be a sign of cancer, particularly colon or uterine cancer.

Fever that accompanies bloating can stem from infection, cancer, or inflammation. If there's also an elevated white blood cell count, infection needs to be immediately excluded, particularly from a pelvic, urinary, or gastrointestinal source.

Ten Diagnoses Linked to Serious Bloating

The three main categories of disease that cause serious bloating are cancer, inflammation, and infection. Cancer is the category most of us worry about the most and is usually the diagnosis you want to definitively diagnose or exclude if you think you may be seriously bloated.

OVARIAN CANCER

This isn't the most likely cause of serious bloating, but it's one of the most lethal, so it's a good idea to familiarize yourself with the symptoms and risk factors. Although ovarian cancer is only the fifth most common cancer in women, it causes more deaths than any other reproductive cancer, mostly in women over fifty. Risk factors include never having children or having them late in life; obesity; a family history of ovarian, breast, or colon cancer; a personal history of breast cancer; certain genetic abnormalities; and long-term treatment with hormone replacement therapy. Bloating, feeling full faster, and pelvic pain are typical symptoms.

Persistent bloating might be particularly worrisome when it comes to ovarian cancer: a British study from 2008 showed that 86 percent of women with ovarian cancer had persistent bloating and distention, whereas only 4.5 percent had fluctuating bloating. A thorough pelvic exam or transvaginal ultrasound, where a probe is inserted into your vagina, is the best way to diagnose ovarian cancer. The blood test CA-125 isn't a reliable screening test but can be helpful for following the course of treatment after diagnosis. Ovarian cancer has sometimes been called the silent killer. It turns out it's not so silent—you just have to know what to listen for.

UTERINE CANCER

Abnormal vaginal bleeding in association with bloating can be a sign of uterine cancer that develops from cells in the lining of the uterus. Other symptoms include a watery or blood-tinged vaginal discharge, pelvic pain, or pain with intercourse or urination. Important risk factors include taking estrogen supplements in the absence of progesterone, tamoxifen, radiation therapy, a family history of uterine cancer, or a family history of a form of inherited colon cancer called Lynch syndrome.

COLON CANCER

Colon cancer can grow to obstruct the inside of the colon and cause progressive bloating. If the cancer is located at the end of the colon in the rectum or sigmoid, there is often bleeding and a history of worsening constipation, but cancers higher up in the colon may initially cause only bloating. Blood in the stool or on the toilet paper should never be ignored. Even if you have hemorrhoids, you still don't know if the blood could be coming from a mass inside your colon, so it needs to be investigated.

Colon cancer is the second most common cause of cancer deaths in nonsmokers in the United States and is mostly preventable through lifestyle changes and regular screening colonoscopies. Some studies have shown that switching to a plant-based, nutrient-rich diet can cut your risk of colon cancer in half. Obesity and belly fat are also risk factors for colon cancer.

PANCREATIC CANCER

This is one of the most dreaded forms of cancer because it tends to be very aggressive and is usually diagnosed in the late stages, so it has a very poor prognosis. The symptoms are nonspecific and include bloating, abdominal pain, and weight loss. A significant percentage of people with pancreatic cancer will develop diabetes a few months before their cancer is diagnosed, and blood clots in the veins may also occur. Bloating associated with painless jaundice, weight loss, loss of appetite, and upper abdominal pain that radiates to the back may indicate pancreatic cancer and is a worrisome constellation of symptoms.

STOMACH CANCER

Stomach cancer is usually asymptomatic early on, or causes vague symptoms like bloating and a feeling of fullness in the upper abdomen. Bloating accompanied by indigestion or heartburn can be an early warning sign. Like pancreatic cancer, it may have already reached an advanced stage at diagnosis, in which case there will likely be additional symptoms of weight loss, nausea, and abdominal pain. Infection with the bacteria *Helicobacter pylori* is felt to be the most important risk factor for the development of stomach cancer, so it's a good idea to be tested for *H. pylori* if you think you may be at risk. The bacterium affects more than half of the world's population, but fortunately it causes symptoms and cancer in only a small percentage of those affected. The nitrates and nitrites in smoked and processed meats are also risk factors, and, in a small number of patients, stomach cancer is genetic.

PERITONEAL CARCINOMATOSIS

Peritoneal carcinomatosis involves widespread dissemination of cancer from a primary site to the lining of the abdominal cavity, often resulting in the production of ascites and a bloated, swollen belly. Ovarian cancer most commonly results in peritoneal carcinomatosis and the prognosis is generally poor.

LIVER DISEASE

Most forms of liver disease are benign, but the liver is also a common site for cancer that spreads from distant organs because when cancer cells get into the bloodstream, they eventually get filtered through the liver. Bloating accompanied by ascites and jaundice may be a sign of cancer that's spread to the liver or of primary liver cancer, which can develop in people with a history of hepatitis or heavy alcohol use.

DIVERTICULITIS

Diverticulitis can cause a combination of bloating, fever, and abdominal pain and is usually accompanied by either diarrhea or constipation (see Chapter 16). The abdomen is tender, especially in the left lower aspect. Bowel rest with a liquid diet is standard treatment, plus antibiotics if there's fever, lots of tenderness, or an elevated white blood cell count. Severe tenderness may prompt your doctor to order a CAT scan to see if you have an abscess, which could require surgical intervention or drainage. Once you've recovered from the acute episode of diverticulitis, a high-fiber diet will help keep you regular and avoid complications.

PELVIC INFLAMMATORY DISEASE

Pelvic inflammatory disease (PID) is caused by infection of the uterine lining, Fallopian tubes, or ovaries, usually from sexually transmitted diseases such as chlamydia and gonorrhea. PID can also occur during childbirth, abortion, or miscarriage, or with insertion of an intrauterine device. Bloating that occurs with fever, pain, and tenderness in the pelvic area plus a vaginal discharge is very suggestive of PID. A pelvic exam and treatment with antibiotics are essential, especially since untreated PID can lead to infertility and ectopic pregnancies (a pregnancy that implants and grows in the Fallopian tubes rather than in the uterus and, if left untreated, can cause life-threatening tubal rupture). Therefore, if you're having bloating, vaginal bleeding or discharge, and lower back or pelvic pain and think you may be pregnant, you should seek immediate medical attention.

CROHN'S DISEASE

Bloating accompanied by fever doesn't always mean infection. Inflammatory conditions such as Crohn's disease can also present this way. Crohn's is an autoimmune digestive disorder that can affect the small intestine or colon. The lag between initial symptoms and diagnosis can be years, and bloating is often one of the early symptoms. Crohn's can cause narrowing of the intestines and ultimately lead to a bowel obstruction, resulting in severe bloating and weight loss, as well as nausea and vomiting after meals. It can also cause bloating in association with diarrhea and blood in the stool. There may be other symptoms present outside of the GI tract, including mouth ulcers, joint pain, skin lesions, and inflammation in the eyes.

I know this hasn't been an easy chapter to read, but the good news is that if you're bloated, you probably don't have cancer, infection, or inflammation, and my 10-Day Gutbliss Plan (see Chapter 23) will probably be all you need to banish your bloat. Nonetheless, it's helpful to know what some of the warning signs and associated symptoms are that might indicate a more worrisome underlying condition, so that you can take the best possible care of yourself. If you're not sure whether you're bloating is serious or not, it's always better to err on the side of seeking medical attention rather than ignoring it and hoping for the best.

PART 3

On the Path to Gutbliss

19

Eating Your Way to Gutbliss

OVER TWO THOUSAND YEARS AGO HIPPOCRATES, THE FATHER OF MOD-
ern medicine, admonished us to "let food be thy medicine and medicine
be thy food." It's advice that's perhaps even more relevant today. Michael
Pollan, my favorite chronicler of where we are nutritionally and how
we got to this sad place, sums it up for us in just seven words: "eat food,
not too much, mostly plants." But where we really need help is with the
word *food*.

My Simple Definition of Food

Much of what I see in the supermarket doesn't meet my simple criteria for
what food really is. Food is supposed to have a beginning, a middle, and
an end. It's something that at some point was alive so, sooner or later, it
should die a natural death.

Food is something that's picked off a tree; plucked from a bush; dug up
from the earth; caught in a river, lake, or ocean; or slaughtered so we can
eat. Putting aside for a moment specifics like whether it's harvested by a
machine or human hand and whether that hand is paid a living wage,
whether it's slaughtered in some secretive and grotesque way, whether it's

full of weird hormones or sprayed with chemicals that can make us sick, whether it's grown in our backyard or on another continent, or whether it's grown at all or just assembled in a laboratory—my basic definition of food is still the same: "something that nourishes us."

Bloating and many of the other digestive ailments I deal with in my practice may be the direct result of our collective departure from "food" as I've just defined it, and the rise of the processed foodstuffs sold in supermarkets, restaurants, and convenience stores today. We've packed our foods with fillers, preservatives, and synthetic vitamins and tampered with the genetic identity of the foods themselves. As you'll see in this chapter, these modifications may be wreaking havoc on our digestive systems and our overall health.

Plenty to Eat, No Food

The food you eat says something about who you are; it can define you just as devoutly as your religion or politics: gluten-free, vegan, locavorian, pescatarian, lacto-ovarian vegetarian, low-carb, or Paleo. People can have very strong opinions about how and what they eat. But the biggest problem I see is not choosing among the different types of diets, but choosing *actual food*. Here in America, we have plenty to eat, but, if you ask me, precious little of it deserves to be called food.

You see this paradox most dramatically at rest stops on any highway or at the gas station, convenience store, or airport: a dizzying array of row after row of edible, food-like substances with expiration dates that stretch on for years and ingredients you've never heard of. Is it possible for something nourishing to have so many chemicals and survive that long on a shelf? *Plenty to eat, no food.*

I keep a number of these edible food-like substances in my drawer at work. I'll often pull out a box and read the ingredients list to patients. Here's what's in a particular brand of animal crackers:

ENRICHED FLOUR (WHEAT FLOUR, NIACIN, REDUCED IRON, THIAMINE MONONITRATE [VITAMIN B_1], RIBOFLAVIN [VITAMIN B_2], FOLIC ACID), HIGH FRUCTOSE CORN SYRUP, SUGAR, SOYBEAN OIL, YELLOW CORN FLOUR, PARTIALLY

HYDROGENATED COTTONSEED OIL, CALCIUM CARBONATE (SOURCE OF CALCIUM), BAKING SODA, SALT, SOY LECITHIN (EMULSIFIER), ARTIFICIAL FLAVOR.

The word *enriched* is usually an indication that the ingredient on its own doesn't have any nutritional value, so they have to add stuff to it. But there's questionable value to adding things like iron and B complex vitamins to food. It's certainly not the same as eating natural sources of these nutrients. There's actually very little convincing data to prove that taking vitamins is of any benefit to our health, either. There are studies that show that people who take vitamins are healthier, but not because of the supplements they take; vitamin users tend to live healthier lifestyles in terms of their habits, including the foods they choose.

You should also be aware that most of the sugar, soy, corn, and cottonseed oil in products like animal crackers is genetically modified, and we're still trying to figure out whether that's a good idea or not. The calcium carbonate listed in the ingredients isn't added to help you build strong bones; it's an anticaking agent that keeps the food from clumping together, and the soy lecithin plays a similar role. I prefer my emulsifiers in paint, not in my food. Then there's the black box of artificial flavor—anyone's guess, since they don't tell you what's in it. These flavors are cheaper to produce and have a longer shelf life than the real thing, but they're often derived from petrochemicals or the paper industry. Not so nourishing.

The time constraints of modern society have made us increasingly unwilling to be inconvenienced by procuring and preparing real food. But when it comes to nutrition, what you put in is directly reflected in what you get out. Today's shortcut food filled with highly processed ingredients and chemicals is undeniably contributing to our declining health, as well as our digestive problems. If I took most parents into the chemistry lab and told them to open up their child's mouth so I could pour beakers filled with food coloring, methylcyclopropene, monosodium glutamate (MSG), sodium benzoate, sodium nitrite, and other commonly used chemicals into their stomachs they'd be horrified and probably call the police. Food for thought.

Addicted to Fake, Hungry for Real

It's no secret why this kind of food can be appealing: it's cheap, accessible, portable, doesn't go bad, and after a while starts to taste pretty good. In fact, we often start to crave it the way we crave drugs and alcohol, which, it turns out, is no coincidence. Neal Barnard, MD, founder of the Physicians Committee for Responsible Medicine, reveals some startling facts about these foods in his book *Breaking the Food Seduction*. Certain foods, sugar in particular, stimulate production of the neurotransmitter dopamine. Dopamine does a lot of things in the brain, chief among them allowing us to feel intense pleasure. Eating lots of sugary foods can create the same effect a drug addict experiences after taking cocaine or heroin—the same dopamine receptors in the brain get stimulated.

Food Then and Now

Our parents and grandparents ate a lot of the same foods we eat—cookies, cakes, sandwiches, casseroles, and maybe even burgers. They probably didn't eat as much of them as we do, but is that the only reason we're generationally so much sicker and more bloated? Or do today's foods have additional features that could be making us ill?

It's possible, if not likely. Most of what we're eating these days has the same cast of characters when it comes to ingredients, at least on paper. But in addition to using much higher amounts of sugar, fat, and salt that appeal to our taste buds, the actual ingredients themselves used in many foods today bear no resemblance to the ones our parents baked and cooked with a generation ago. Much of our corn, soy, sugar, canola, and cottonseed oils (as well as some produce like tomatoes, potatoes, papaya, and squash) has been altered through a process of genetic modification. Genetic modification takes the genetic material from one organism and inserts it into the permanent genetic code of another, creating novel substances such as potatoes with bacteria genes, pigs with human genes, and fish with cattle genes. It's estimated that more than 70 percent of processed foods on supermarket shelves today contain genetically engineered ingredients.

Flying on Empty

Anyone who travels has probably spent more time than they'd like hanging around airports. Consequently, it's where I do some of my most eyebrow-raising food sleuthing. Most airport foods are prime examples of being nothing more than sugar molecules rearranged differently. That can add up to a whole lot of not-very-nutritious pleasure while you try to ignore the pain of your delayed flight.

Besides sugar, other ingredients in airport food can be equally addictive:

- MSG is known for causing headaches but also makes us feel hungry a short time after eating.
- Salt desensitizes our taste buds so we start to add more and more of it to our food.
- Cheese contains casein and casomorphins, both of which both have opiate effects.
- Eating flour begets eating more flour.
- Fat is filling and therefore satisfies our evolutionary tendency to eat calorie-rich food, even if it's nutrient-poor.

People whose diets consist primarily of airport-type food tend to be overweight but undernourished. Despite taking in way more than enough calories, they're still missing essential vitamins and nutrients, so they keep on eating. It's a vicious cycle of insatiable hunger, yet starvation for actual food. These foods elicit typical addict behavior, likely related to the dopamine effects: indulgence and pleasure, accompanied by tolerance, followed by withdrawal, triggering the whole cycle to repeat over and over. Who ever thought that food could be so harmful?

There are advantages and disadvantages to genetic modification. Potential benefits include enhanced nutrient content, improved taste, resistance to pathogens and disease, increased crop yield, enhanced shelf life, and food that is cheaper to grow. The downside is that nature is an incredibly complex system of interconnected species, and many scientists worry about the long-term risks, as well as unintended and irreversible consequences of tampering with that process. Concerns about genetic modification fall into three main categories: health risks to humans, damage to the environment, and the economic consequences of corporations controlling the food supply through access to seeds.

The Center for Food Safety is a nonprofit public interest and environmental advocacy organization established in 1997 to challenge what it views as harmful food production technologies and to promote sustainable alternatives. It maintains that genetically engineered foods may pose serious health risks to humans, including higher risks of toxicity and allergenicity.

Monsanto is a multinational agricultural biotech company founded in 1901 and the leading producer of genetically engineered seeds. It maintains that so long as the genetically introduced protein is determined safe, food from genetically modified (GM) crops is not expected to pose any health risks. Long-term safety testing of GM foods in humans is cumbersome and not readily available, as it would require ingesting large amounts of a particular GM product over an extended period of time. But there is a large body of documented scientific testing under the auspices of the Center for Environmental Risk Assessment (CERA) that shows that currently authorized GM crops are safe.

CERA is part of the International Life Sciences Institute (ILSI). ILSI is a nonprofit organization founded in 1978, the members of which are primarily food and beverage, agricultural, chemical, and pharmaceutical companies, and ILSI receives funding mainly from those members.

Notwithstanding the CERA studies documenting the nutritional value of GM crops and the safety of the modifications used, there may be an inherent conflict of interest when companies with billions of dollars at stake are the ones responsible for reporting the safety of their own products. We've seen how this can go awry in the pharmaceutical industry, which has considerably more regulation in place: the odds of research coming to a conclusion favorable to a drug are 3.6 times greater when funded by the company making the drug.

Although from a scientific point of view I recognize the potential benefits of genetic modification, I can't help but be wary of GM foods, not least because, as a gastroenterologist, I've watched so many new and chronic digestive complaints pop up since their mainstream introduction in the late 1990s. The biggest increase is in the area of food allergies, food intolerances, and microscopic inflammation in the gut. While this certainly doesn't prove cause and effect, it's worth considering what the long-term effects of consuming these foods in large amounts might be.

UNFORTUNATELY, NOT SCIENCE FICTION

Here's just one example of how these products could be contributing to your bloating.

Bacillus thuringiensis, otherwise known as Bt, is a hardy and clever bacterium that lives in soil and creates its own insecticide—the Bt toxin—that kills insects by making their stomachs burst open. The insecticide works by creating holes in the membranes of cells in the insects' guts. Biotech companies have inserted the gene for Bt toxin into corn so that it can produce its own insecticide. The idea was that the toxin would kill the insects but be completely destroyed in our digestive system, so that it wouldn't pose a threat to human health. But along the way, something rather unexpected happened: a Canadian study in 2011 found that the Bt toxin that was supposed to be destroyed in our gut was actually present in 93 percent of pregnant women tested, 80 percent of umbilical blood in their babies, and 67 percent of nonpregnant women.

Bt corn is in almost all processed food and drinks through the widespread use of high fructose corn syrup. It's also in meat, since most meat comes from livestock fed Bt corn on factory farms or CAFOs (concentrated animal feeding operations—you can tell from the name, which does not have a nice ring to it, that life on a CAFO for the average cow is not fun). Other studies have confirmed that the genes inserted into genetically engineered foods can be transferred to our gut bacteria. So instead of being destroyed, the Bt toxin may actually be present and continually produced by organisms in our digestive tract.

Leaky gut syndrome is a relatively new and not entirely understood problem (see Chapter 14, "Could Your Gut Be Leaking?"). Some in the medical community believe leaky gut is the underlying mechanism behind many of the allergic and inflammatory digestive problems that we're seeing in such high numbers. Remember those holes in the membranes of cells in the insects' guts? Well, in humans with leaky gut, the junctions between cells in the lining of the intestine literally start to leak, allowing substances to enter the bloodstream that normally couldn't go through the membrane—a phenomenon we call increased intestinal permeability.

Normally the intestinal lining acts as a very selective strainer with tiny holes, allowing certain nutrients and well-digested food particles of a limited size to go through and keeping out larger viruses, bacteria, and toxins. When the gut becomes inflamed and leaky, bigger molecules, including large particles of food that aren't properly broken down and digested, are able to go through the damaged strainer and enter the bloodstream. The immune system tends to freak out when this happens. It's not used to seeing these large particles of various foods, and the result is allergic reactions.

In my practice, I see people with allergies to almost every kind of food, not just the common things like nuts or milk. My patients often have unusual symptoms, such as flushing, bloating, and swelling soon after eating, and with lots of different foods. In the typical person with an intact digestive membrane, being allergic to so many foods would be highly unusual. When you think of someone with a leaky gut, however, it makes perfect sense.

Leaky gut doesn't just cause increased intestinal permeability and allergic reactions; it also decreases nutrient absorption by the villi, the millions of tiny, fingerlike projections in the small intestine. So even if you're eating a healthy, balanced diet, the absorption of the vitamins and minerals you desperately need for good health is decreased, while the absorption of the undigested food particles and bad bugs is increased. Leaky gut is also associated with overgrowth of undesirable bacterial species and yeast, whose by-products include large amounts of bloat-causing methane gas.

Italian scientists have found a wide range of immune responses in mice fed Bt corn, including elevated antibodies, cytokines, and T cells of the kind typically associated with allergic and autoimmune reactions. This has led researchers to wonder whether the dramatic increase we're seeing in allergic and inflammatory conditions could be related to some of these engineered substances that are arguably not meant for human consumption.

I wonder about the same thing in many of my patients with irritable bowel syndrome, inflammatory conditions, food allergies, and unexplained bloating. Their symptoms frequently seem to be correlated with something they're eating, but we just can't put our finger on what it is. As I noted in Chapter 14, some of them describe feeling "poisoned." Invariably they feel better when they avoid food altogether but, of course, that's not a long-term solution. Spray insecticides can be washed off our food, but genetically inserted toxins like Bt, in addition to being modified from their naturally occurring state, are part of the food we eat—they can't be separated or avoided.

In 2010 the American Academy of Environmental Medicine recommended that physicians tell their patients to exclude genetically modified foods from their diets. Like many other organizations, it also called for more independent, long-term safety studies and the labeling of foods that contain genetically modified ingredients. We're still learning about the long-term effects of genetic modification of our food. My approach for patients with bloating, inflammation, food allergies, food intolerances, or autoimmune conditions is to recommend excluding these foods from their diet—not because there is a clear link but because there might be.

My patient Sheila was well until two years ago, when she suddenly developed redness, itching, and swelling of her face and hands, which went away after a few hours. She saw a rheumatologist who thought it was an allergic reaction, but her labs came back showing a positive blood test for lupus, an autoimmune disease that can affect many different organ systems, including the joints, skin, kidneys, blood cells, lungs, and heart. She had no real signs of lupus at the time—no chronic skin rashes, joint pain or swelling, kidney problems, fever, fatigue, or anemia. Given the lack of physical complaints, they decided to watch her closely and recheck her labs in a few months.

During that time Sheila started to develop relentless bloating and diarrhea after every meal. At her follow-up visit with the rheumatologist, the lupus test was even more abnormal, so a prescription drug called Plaquenil was recommended, and she was referred to me for evaluation of the diarrhea.

Before coming to see me Sheila did some research on lupus and decided to put herself on an anti-inflammatory diet. She eliminated gluten, dairy, sugar, soy, and meat and shifted to a plant-based diet plus a little organic chicken and fish. Within about two weeks her diarrhea improved, and she was no longer having accidents and soiling herself. Her lupus blood test was much improved, too, although still abnormal. However, she was still feeling bloated after most meals, and her stools still weren't fully formed.

Since she had given up wheat and most animal protein, Sheila was now eating a lot of corn products—chips, tortillas, popcorn, and corn flour baked goods. We eliminated the corn, and her bloating and stools normalized within about a month. And most interesting, by her next rheumatology visit, the blood work for lupus was normal, too.

Sheila eventually stopped the Plaquenil but remained on the diet and has continued to feel well. It's unclear whether she ever really had lupus, but something was definitely awry with her immune system and her gut, and the dietary changes were tremendously helpful in getting things back to normal. I've had lots of patients respond favorably to an anti-inflammatory diet that removes most processed grains, refined sugars, and other GM foods, with visible improvement of gut inflammation, symptoms, and blood tests. My 10-Day Gutbliss Plan (see Chapter 23) isn't as drastic as what Sheila ultimately embarked on, but it certainly gets you started on the path to healing inflammation and banishing bloat.

It's easy to become disconnected from food these days, when so few of us are involved in growing, harvesting, or even cooking the food we eat. But it's impossible to separate what we're eating from how we're feeling, since we truly are what we eat (and what our food eats, too!). I'm not suggesting that changing your diet is the solution for everyone, but it is worth seriously considering whether the food you're eating could be contributing to your digestive problems—a notion that seems intuitive to me as a gastroenterologist but is still not accepted by many in the medical community. We're still learning about conditions like leaky gut, food allergies, and autoimmune diseases, but my hunch is that in the years to come, we'll have even more evidence that most diseases have their origin in the gut and that food can be our best medicine, as well as our worst poison.

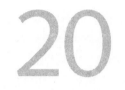

Drinking Your Way to Gutbliss

WE DON'T ALWAYS PAY AS MUCH ATTENTION TO WHAT WE'RE DRINK-
ing as we do to what we're eating. You may think that as long as you're
drinking something, you're hydrating yourself, regardless of what that
something is. Liquids are essential for moving the products of digestion
smoothly through the intestines, but if you're drinking the wrong ones,
you could actually be causing dehydration and bloating. Some liquids are
also very calorie dense, which can lead to rapid weight gain. In this chapter you'll learn about some of the biggest offenders when it comes to what
I call the "potable bloatables." I'll also recommend alternatives that can
reduce your bloat, hydrate you, and keep your intestinal contents moist
and moving.

The Potable Bloatables

DAIRY

Dairy is one of the biggest contributors of fat to the American diet, much
of it in the form of milk. There are three main reasons why I don't recommend dairy if you're bloated or having gastrointestinal issues, regardless
of whether it's full cream, skim, or low-fat:

1. lactose intolerance,
2. pasteurization, and
3. hormones.

Lactose Intolerance

More than half the world's population has some degree of lactose intolerance. That means the small intestine doesn't make enough of the enzyme lactase, which you need to digest lactose, the sugar present in milk. Lactose intolerance can develop anytime from infancy to adulthood. It can be tricky to diagnose because the symptoms overlap with other conditions such as irritable bowel syndrome (IBS) and celiac disease, which can also cause bloating, diarrhea, gas, and abdominal cramping.

When I think a patient might have lactose intolerance, my first step is to recommend an avoidance trial: avoiding any and all dairy for a minimum of a week to see if symptoms improve. (A lactose hydrogen breath test is a more formal way of diagnosing lactose intolerance, but it's more cumbersome than simply assessing a patient's symptoms after a week of avoidance.) In someone who is lactose-intolerant, lactose passes undigested from the small intestine to the colon, where it undergoes fermentation by bacteria into hydrogen and other gases. A rise in the level of these gases detected during the breath test is considered evidence of lactase deficiency.

Once the diagnosis is made, some people choose to continue to eliminate dairy products from their diet as a way of controlling their symptoms. Those with milder symptoms or who consider the dietary change a hardship may be able to get away with small amounts of yogurt and hard cheeses, which contain less lactose than things like ice cream and mozzarella. Most people with low lactase levels can tolerate small amounts of dairy but will have symptoms with larger doses. I generally don't recommend using lactase supplements or products with added lactase on a regular basis, because if your body can't digest something, avoidance rather than repeated exposure seems like the more sensible approach.

Lactose intolerance is common, but it can also be a sign of other problems in the GI tract. Celiac disease and Crohn's can both cause lactose intolerance because of damage to the lining of the small intestine where the enzyme lactase is secreted. Temporary or permanent lactose intolerance can occur with giardia and rotavirus infection. For patients with nausea, vomiting, or diarrhea suggestive of a "stomach bug," I'll usually advise that they avoid dairy and then cautiously reintroduce it once the acute illness is over.

If you think you might be lactose intolerant, there's no harm in doing an avoidance trial, but if your symptoms don't completely resolve after eliminating dairy, then by all means seek medical advice to make sure you don't have an underlying gastrointestinal condition like IBS, celiac disease, Crohn's, or an infection.

Pasteurization

We've been pasteurizing milk for well over a hundred years to decrease spoilage from bacteria and extend its shelf life. The process involves heating the milk to very high temperatures, then rapidly cooling it. The problem with pasteurization is that it also destroys lots of the naturally occurring beneficial bacteria and vitamins in milk. Some alternative health practitioners recommend raw, unpasteurized dairy as a source of beneficial bacteria, but it will still cause problems if you're lactose intolerant.

Hormones

Hormones that are used to increase milk production in some commercial dairy cows may have an estrogen-like effect, which can in turn lead to a condition called estrogen dominance. Estrogen dominance, which I discuss in Chapter 8, "What's Happening with Your Hormones?," is what occurs when estrogen is disproportionately elevated relative to progesterone. Estrogen dominance is a major cause of bloating and can worsen other conditions that contribute to bloating, such as fibroids and endometriosis.

SODA

No one would argue that soda is health food or part of a nutritious diet, but you may not realize that it's a major cause of bloating. Sweeteners in soda are usually sugar, high fructose corn syrup, or poorly absorbed carbohydrates like maltodextrin or artificial sweeteners. The high sugar content (almost ten teaspoons in some brands!) can lead to bloating from overgrowth of undesirable bacterial species and yeast, especially candida, which feed on sugar, not to mention the extra weight a daily soda can lead to—54,750 calories a year, which equals fifteen pounds.

Some studies have shown that artificial sweeteners cause a spike in insulin—a hormone associated with fat storage, diabetes, and inflammation—and although they may be low-calorie, they can cause just as much weight gain as regular soda.

And finally, poorly absorbed (nonnutritive) carbohydrates and artificial sweeteners don't get broken down and digested in the small intestine, so they undergo a lot of fermentation by colonic bacteria, leading to gas and bloating. Bloating can also be a result of undiagnosed fructose intolerance, and soda sweetened with fructose can greatly contribute to those symptoms.

SPORTS DRINKS

Unlike soda, these drinks are often marketed as being healthy and full of important electrolytes, but unless you're training for an Ironman triathlon, you probably don't need the extra sodium and other salts—unless, that is, you're trying to add to your bloat. The sugar and other sweeteners in these products have the same effect as soda, contributing to bacterial overgrowth and weight gain. Most people don't pay attention to how many calories they're consuming when they drink sports drinks because they're lured in by the health claims. In many cases the calories consumed far exceed the calories burned at the gym. The best way to hydrate after a workout is with water. If you're worried about electrolytes, eat a banana.

FRUIT JUICE

Like soda, fruit juices can contain a lot of sugar or fructose, so they can also cause bacterial overgrowth, problems with candida, bloating from fructose intolerance, and weight gain. In a recent study from the University of Kansas, almost half of all normal people who were exposed to fructose experienced gas. You may think you're making a healthy choice by choosing fruit juice over soda, but the sugar content in juice can be even higher than in soda. Labeling that claims no added sugar can be misleading because there's often already a very high naturally occurring sugar content. If you have bacterial imbalance in your gut, the additional sugar can lead to tremendous bloating because the bacteria and yeast species thrive on it. And unlike a piece of fruit, there's no fiber in fruit juice to slow down the body's absorption of sugar, leading to a spike in insulin release.

ALCOHOL

Alcohol causes bloating in a number of ways. Alcohol made from gluten-containing grains like wheat and barley can be irritating to the lining of the small intestine if you have celiac disease or are gluten intolerant. Alcohol can also irritate the lining of the stomach, causing a condition called gastritis where the protective mucus layer is stripped away, leaving the stomach vulnerable to the effects of stomach acid and digestive enzymes. Alcoholic gastritis can lead to severe bloating and abdominal discomfort.

Alcohol can also add lots of pounds to your waistline. It's converted to acetate in the liver, which slows the body's fat-burning processes. In addition, while under the influence of alcohol, many of us will make poor food choices, which, along with the empty alcohol calories, can really add pounds.

Last but not least, alcohol is dehydrating, which can cause electrolyte shifts that bloat our abdomens and give us an overall puffy, swollen appearance.

CAFFEINE

Since caffeine can be a diuretic, you might think it would help with bloating, but it turns out that caffeine can actually contribute to bloating. Caffeinated beverages, especially coffee, can stimulate the digestive system, leading to spasms that can cause bloating. Caffeine can also worsen conditions associated with bloating, such as stomach ulcers, gastritis, and IBS. Decaffeinated beverages have also been associated with some of these symptoms. Despite the stimulant effect of caffeine, which can trigger bowel movements in some people, the diuretic effect can lead to dehydration, slowing down movement through the intestines and causing backups and bloating.

SOY MILK

For people who are lactose intolerant, a soy latte may seem like a good idea, but processed soy can be a big contributor to your bloat. In Asia, small amounts of unprocessed fermented soy like miso, natto, and tempeh have been associated with health benefits, primarily from encouraging the growth of beneficial bacterial species. But large amounts of processed unfermented soy, as are commonly used in the West in place of dairy or as filler in foods, can have the opposite result: estrogen-like effects, which contribute to bloating, weight gain, and symptoms of estrogen dominance. Additionally, soy can slow down thyroid function and trigger thyroid disease in some individuals, which is a major cause of bloating.

CARBONATED DRINKS

I prefer fizzy water to flat, but when I'm bloated I definitely avoid carbonation. Dissolving carbon dioxide in water creates carbonic acid, which gives fizzy water its bubbles and leaves you with a bloated stomach full of carbon dioxide gas. Bottled or canned carbonated water may also contain sodium and other salts that are added to enhance the taste, and the additional salt can further contribute to the bloating effect.

KOMBUCHA

Kombucha is a drink made by fermenting kombucha culture, which consists of bacteria and yeast mixed with sugar and water. Although considered by many to be a detoxifying agent, the health claims tend to be much exaggerated, and some people consuming kombucha products on a regular basis have problems with bloating. Although the manufacturers claim that some of the yeast species are helpful, it's difficult to predict the exact microbial content of different batches. Bacterial contamination when kombucha is brewed at home is also a concern.

What Should You Be Drinking?

If it seems as if I've taken all your liquids away, don't worry; there's still lots to drink that won't cause bloating and may even help it.

WATER

Clearly the liquid you should be drinking the most of is water. More than half of our body consists of water, and since there are so many factors in daily life that cause dehydration, from medications to caffeine to heaters to air conditioners to simply not enough intake, you need to be sure you're replenishing your body's water supply. Drinking lots of water is one of the best things you can do to banish bloating. Water promotes good digestion, keeping the intestines moist and the contents moving briskly, which prevents bloat-causing backups and constipation. I recommend at least a liter a day, although the requirement will vary based on the climate you live in, how hydrating or dehydrating the rest of your diet is, and what your fluid losses are.

COCONUT WATER

I'm a huge fan of coconut water, which in its pure form contains relatively small amounts of sugar, no preservatives, and sufficient naturally occurring electrolytes such as potassium to help combat dehydration. I've kept many patients who were suffering from infectious gastroenteritis or colitis flares out of the hospital by using coconut water as rehydration therapy. Coconut water is a great alternative to soda or sugary fruit juices, but it isn't a low-calorie drink, so you still need to be mindful of how much you're consuming, or the calories and sugar can start to add up.

HERBAL TEAS

Most herbal teas are naturally caffeine free and are a great alternative to coffee or caffeinated teas. The water you use to brew them can count toward the liter a day I recommend. Just make sure you're not adding heaps of milk and sugar, which can add calories and encourage bloat. You may like your tea hot, but many of the herbal and fruit infusions have a refreshing tartness that is also cooling and tasty in iced tea.

GREEN JUICES AND SMOOTHIES

My favorite way to hydrate is a little labor-intensive but well worth it: green juices and smoothies. There's no wrong or right way to make them, as long as you're using well-washed and preferably organic produce and not overdoing it with the fruit. You'll need a juicer for the green juices and a strong blender for the smoothies—for recipes to get you started, see my 10-Day Gutbliss Plan in Chapter 23. My absolute favorite green juice is kale, spinach, and green apple. For smoothies, I love blending berries,

Gutbliss Solutions for Developing Fluid Habits

What liquids you drink tends to be habit more than anything else, especially when it comes to coffee and soda.

Getting soda of any kind out of your diet is one of the healthiest things you can do, and one of the most helpful in terms of bloating.

You may be able to get away with a limited amount of caffeine, like a cup a day. But remember, a cup is 8 ounces, not the oversized containers on offer from your friendly neighborhood barista. Beware of caffeine creep, since it tends to be addictive and you eventually develop a tolerance. Also, try not to turn your coffee or tea into a milk shake with tons of milk and sugar.

Get in the habit of drinking more water—at least a liter a day—by identifying convenient times to drink it and scheduling it into your day. It may be during your daily commute, or between dinner and bedtime when you're at home and the bathroom is nearby.

When you need some flavor and plain water just won't do, add a splash of fruit juice to carbonated water for a spritzer if the bubbles don't bother you, or use flat water with a ratio of four parts water to one part juice and some ice.

Use electrolyte-rich coconut water as a rehydration solution, but don't overdo it since the sugar and calories can add up.

Try a green juice or fruit and veggie smoothie for hydration plus lots of nutrients. See the 10-Day Gutbliss Plan in Chapter 23 and the Recipes section (see Appendix) for my favorite recipes.

Experiment with either hot or cold caffeine-free herbal teas.

---

bananas, and almond milk with shredded collard greens, spinach, or kale. Add some ground flax seed or psyllium husk for an additional anti-bloating boost. Be wary of premade, commercially sold smoothies and juices. Despite the healthy names, many of them have large amounts of sugar from apple juice, other sweet fruit, or even added sweeteners, and little in the way of green vegetables. Some of the popular brands sold in supermarkets have way more sugar than a serving of ice cream.

Remember that bloating is often a sign that what you're eating or drinking isn't agreeing with you, or that things are backed up along your digestive superhighway. Paying attention to your liquid intake can be an essential part of banishing your bloat—keeping you well hydrated and your digestive contents moist and moving.

21

On the Move Toward Gutbliss

LAST YEAR I SIGNED UP TO BE A MEDICAL VOLUNTEER AT THE IRONMAN championship in Kona, Hawaii. Competing at Kona is on my bucket list, but I'm not quite there (okay, I'm not even close), so the next best thing was working in the medical tent. I was curious to see what sort of condition people would be in after swimming 2.4 miles, biking 112 miles, and then running 26.2 miles in one-hundred-degree heat.

Most of the competitors I tended to in the medical tent that night were simply dehydrated and exhausted. We weigh the athletes before the race, and a few had lost ten pounds or more. Many hobbled in with painful muscle spasms, and one had to be sent to the hospital for pulmonary edema—lungs full of water instead of air. Some had been swimming, riding, and running for seventeen hours (the cutoff for being pulled off the course if you haven't completed all 140.6 miles by midnight). It was incredible and inspiring to witness what my fellow human beings were capable of.

My observation after the race was that there are three kinds of people: über-athletes such as the Ironman competitors, couch potatoes, and those of us in between. My time spent in and around the digestive tract suggests three categories there, too: bowel movements that are so precise you can set your clock to their arrival, ones that are perennially tardy and sometimes stand you up altogether, and those in between. Which kind of bathroom habits you have may also reflect what kind of training you've been doing, both to maintain your GI regularity and to stay active in general—although fortunately it doesn't take swimming, cycling, and running all day to whip your intestines into shape, and, of course, there are other factors beyond exercise that determine bowel activity. Still, the fact is that your digestive tract is one long muscle, and if you're not moving, chances are your bowels aren't, either.

The Workout Within

The smooth muscles that make up the long, hollow intestinal tube both propel and mix digested food as it travels. This movement, known as peristalsis, consists of wavelike motions as the muscles contract and relax and the products of digestion are moved efficiently through the system. The intestinal muscles are arranged in layers: circular muscles alternating with longitudinal ones. Contraction of the circular muscles initiates the peristaltic wave, while subsequent longitudinal contractions provide the propulsion. Earthworms use a similar peristaltic system for their locomotion.

The GI tract is mostly smooth muscle, which contracts involuntarily, unlike the biceps and hamstrings, which are skeletal muscles under voluntary control that can be directed by us to contract or relax. So, if the muscular contractions of peristalsis happen involuntarily, what's the connection between physical activity and gastrointestinal fitness? Well, despite the fact that peristalsis occurs without our effort or consciousness, our level of physical activity does have an impact on the involuntary muscle contraction of our GI tract. In fact, exercise is one of the most important stimulators of peristalsis:

- Exercise decreases transit time through the entire digestive tract so that your stools arrive at their final destination faster.
- Gravitational forces at work during exercise help to propel the stool downward toward the rectum.
- Exercise increases production of nitric oxide, a chemical that relaxes the smooth muscles of the digestive tract and speeds up peristalsis.

We've learned from our cardiology colleagues that nitric oxide is essential to vascular health. It relaxes the blood vessels that feed the heart, boosting blood flow and preventing the buildup of plaque that can cause heart attacks. It has a similar protective effect in the GI tract by keeping the mucosa healthy and preventing white blood cells that mediate inflammation from sticking to the lining.

- Exercise can greatly increase lymphatic flow. Lymphatic fluid is a sort of bath that surrounds our cells, transporting digested fats and metabolic waste through the body. Poor lymphatic flow can lead to bloating.
- Vigorous bouncing-type exercises like horseback riding, running, and some forms of yoga have been shown to increase the output of bile from the liver, which can enhance digestion and decrease bloating.
- Physical activity decreases cholesterol levels in bile. High levels of cholesterol in bile contribute to the formation of gallstones—hard, pebble-like deposits that form inside the gallbladder.
- Exercise is a potent tool for treating constipation and bloating, and runners actually have better bowel movements: not as hard, bigger, and more frequent.

Over and over, I've observed that my most active patients tend to have fewer GI problems and much less bloating. In contrast, bedbound, sedentary patients can develop such severe bloating and constipation that someone has to manually remove the stool from their colon, an unpleasant task for both parties called fecal disempaction.

There's lots of scientific evidence to support this inverse relationship between exercise and the likelihood of developing digestive problems, including cancer, gallstones, diverticulosis, constipation, reflux, and certain types of inflammation:

- Exercise can decrease the risk of colon cancer by up to 25 percent, independent of other risk factors like diet and weight.
- Two clinical trials showed that colon cancer survivors who exercised regularly extended their life span. The likely mechanism is that exercise speeds up transit time through the intestines, which limits the amount of time cancer-causing toxins are in contact with it.
- Other factors that increase the risk of colon cancer all improved with

exercise, adding to exercise's protective effect. Among these risks are a high body mass index (BMI) indicative of obesity; insulin resistance, where your cells don't respond to the normal actions of insulin, the chemical that brings glucose (your body's main energy nutrient) to your cells; and elevated triglyceride levels in the blood from a high-fat diet.

- A European study published in 2010 revealed that people with gall-stones who were physically active had fewer symptoms than their sedentary counterparts, and the overall risk reduction was as much as 70 percent in the most active group. These beneficial effects seem to be synergistic with nutritional modifications such as a high-fiber, low-fat diet.

- Studies show that exercise can both prevent gallstones from forming and reduce symptoms if you already have them.

- Jogging and running have been shown in clinical studies to reduce the risk of diverticulosis by increasing colonic activity, enhancing transit times through the colon, improving blood flow, and decreasing pressure within the colon.

- Even elderly people can benefit from exercise: research shows an improvement in bowel movement patterns as well as a decrease in lax-ative use in elderly patients participating in a combined exercise and nutrition program, even with low-intensity exercise. A little bit of movement can go a long way in terms of bowel function.

Delayed emptying of the stomach, a condition called gastroparesis (which I discussed in Chapter 3), makes you particularly prone to bloat-ing. Fortunately, exercise can significantly improve gastric emptying in most people. A brisk evening walk after dinner can help to move things along and is a great alternative to the after-dinner TV slump, which can slow things down even more. With delayed gastric emptying it's impor-tant to be mindful of avoiding overly vigorous exercise too soon after eat-ing, when the stomach might still be full. A brisk walk will help, but a fast run right after eating might cause indigestion. If you have slow emptying, waiting at least four hours after a meal before vigorous exercise will help you boost peristalsis without the discomfort of a full stomach.

From a gastrointestinal point of view, the hazards of exercise are few.

Although intense exercise for long periods of time has been known to cause nausea, heartburn, diarrhea, and, rarely, gastrointestinal bleeding, these symptoms are almost always limited to very extreme exercise and may even be considered protective by forcing you to slow down or stop if you're overdoing it.

Choosing Your Exercise

If you ask me what kind of exercise you should be doing, I'll tell you that just as there are no bad vegetables, there really are no bad forms of exercise. Some are more dangerous, or require more skill or lots of fancy equipment, but I can't think of any that I would recommend you avoid, with the caveat of proper hydration, adequate nutrition, listening to your body, warming up, et cetera. I'm a yogi and a runner, and I also enjoy spinning (indoor cycling) classes, so I'm going to go into a little bit more detail about how those forms of exercise can be helpful with bloating.

The emotional and spiritual benefits of yoga have been well described, and I can definitely vouch for feeling cleansed and renewed after my heated Vinyasa flow class. For anyone who's ever done a downward-facing dog, the gastrointestinal benefits of yoga aren't hard to believe. Yoga is sort of a twofer: it can relieve stress as well as the actual physical symptoms of many digestive disorders. That's in part due to the strengthening of the core abdominal muscles, which help to bind the intestines in place and prevent bulging and bloating. The belly breathing techniques in some forms of yoga can provide powerful pain relief, and the twisting poses can help improve gas and constipation. Gas tends to get trapped in two places along the digestive tract: the left upper corner of the abdomen, where the spleen can press on the bowels, and the right upper corner, where the liver can do the same thing. Poses that involve twisting at the waist can help to disperse those gas pockets and relieve pressure.

Some of the intestinal benefit is purely mechanical—things moving through better—and some of it may be related to stimulation of the lymphatic and endocrine systems, as well as optimized hormone secretion. Studies show that yoga can raise levels of the feel-good hormone serotonin as well as endorphins, and decrease stress-related hormones like cortisol, improving both mood and bloating.

Claims that yoga helps to stimulate the adrenal glands and detoxify the kidneys may be more difficult to prove. The reality is we're not exactly sure of the specific mechanisms for how yoga works to help the body, and we don't have lots of scientific studies to prove some of the theories about the benefits of yoga. But the huge number of people doing yoga regularly (fifteen million in the United States alone) suggests that it's doing something helpful.

If you read through the psychiatric literature, you'll find a lot of articles about long-distance runners getting depressed when they stop running. If you examine this phenomenon carefully, what becomes clear is that for many it's not the absence of exercise that's causing their depression; it's the presence of exercise that's treating it. Many people have somehow, consciously or subconsciously, figured out that running and other forms of exercise improve their mood and keep their depression under good control. I've seen the same phenomenon in runners who develop constipation and bloating after an injury sidelines them. For many, a daily run is their foolproof guarantee of satisfaction in the bathroom and a bloat-free existence.

We've already discussed some of the physiologic benefits of exercise, and virtually all of them apply to running, but there are additional features of this form of exercise that can help bloating symptoms. Running burns about 100 calories every ten minutes, assuming a ten-minute-per-mile pace. For most of us, that sort of expenditure will also cause us to sweat—a great way to remove toxins via what I like to think of as the external GI tract—the skin. When we sweat, we tend to drink more water. More water is one of the fundamental rules for improving bloating: it improves motility, lymphatic flow, stool consistency, and regularity. There are few other times during the day when we would consider downing a liter bottle of water in one sitting. If you're careful not to consume more calories than you burn (and by this I mean you should avoid things like sports drinks and flavored waters, which can be as much as 150 calories and loaded with sugars, artificial sweeteners, and other chemicals—see Chapter 20, "Drinking Your Way to Gutbliss," for details) and to replace all the fluids you've lost and then some, running can translate to extra hydration, which does a bloated body good. Plus, it's convenient, free, doesn't require special equipment (a good bra/athletic supporter, maybe, but not even special sneakers anymore), can be done anywhere, including jogging on the spot if you can't get outdoors and don't have a treadmill, and can be enjoyed by people of all ages (unlike their more sedentary counterparts, the senior citizens I know who are runners spend far more time talking about miles logged than their bowel habits). Running on un- paved roads or trails, and mixing in other forms of exercise such as walk- ing and swimming, which put less stress on your lower body, can help to protect your joints and extend your running career.

Spinning is a group cycling workout done on a stationary bike and an excellent way to burn calories, relieve stress, increase cardiovascular fit- ness, and avoid excessive pressure on the joints while building muscle tone in the lower extremities. It can also strengthen abdominal and pelvic floor muscles, which can be an essential part of developing more effective elimination and less bloating. One of the local spinning studios that I frequent has a dimly lit spinning room with candles that helps to create a soothing atmosphere, a high-energy soundtrack, and instructors that make the class feel more like a dance party than a workout. It's a winning combination that for many of my patients leads to improved regularity not just at the spinning studio, but in the bathroom, too.

There's an almost endless variety of exercise options to suit every age and fitness level: swimming, martial arts, kickboxing, ballet, bicycling, spin class, weight training, aerobics, Pilates, brisk walking, and all man- ner of sports, from tennis to volleyball to baseball to soccer, and many more. If you're new to exercise or haven't been exercising regularly, start slowly and work your way up, gradually increasing your stamina and strength to avoid injury that can sideline and discourage you. Make sure you're supporting your activity level with adequate hydration, balanced nutrition, and a sound training plan.

I would thoroughly and without reservation recommend that regular exercise in whatever manner appeals to you be a part of your gutbliss journey, letting your body encourage you to do more and tell you when you've had enough. It's good at that. Whether it's low-tech or complex, away from home or done in your living room, super-affordable or pricey, with others or on your own, exercise is great for your guts.

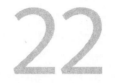

Beauty and the Bloat

ALTHOUGH BLOATING IS ONE OF THE MOST COMMON COMPLAINTS I SEE
in my gastroenterology practice, it might surprise you to know that hair
loss and skin problems are also at the top of the list. People frequently
wonder if there's a nutritional component to why they're losing hair or
having cystic acne in their thirties and forties, so they come in for a con-
sult to see if the problem could be in their gut. And it often is, although it
may be more complicated than food alone. When it comes to your appearance, your GI tract might actually play a bigger role than your genes, because without healthy bowels, it's really hard to have glowing skin or a full
head of hair. Your digestive tract is like the soil, and your hair and skin are
like the plants: if the soil isn't healthy, the plants won't bloom properly.
The good news is that the combination of bad skin, thinning hair, and a
bloated belly often has one unifying cause, and treating it often improves
all three conditions.

In this chapter we'll look at the gut-based problems behind many common skin and hair conditions and what to do about them. I'll give you my
take on cleansing and detoxification, and some essential tips for banishing bloat on the inside and creating a healthy glow on the outside. I'll also

share some amazing recipes for edible skin and hair-care products straight from the kitchen.

Before we get started, let me point out that some of the hypotheses about gut-skin interaction I'm going to discuss are just that: hypothetical. We don't know precisely what causes skin conditions such as acne, rosacea, and eczema, and there are probably multiple factors involved. But it seems logical and likely that the gut plays a significant role, since inflammation in the skin is often a reaction to substances that enter the body through the digestive tract. While I'm very qualified to diagnose and treat digestive problems, I'm not a dermatologist. My comments here represent a combination of what is known from the scientific literature and my own observations about skin and hair problems in the many patients with GI problems I've seen over the years.

The Gut-Skin Connection

When a patient walks into my office, I can see what's going on with her skin far more quickly than what might be happening in her digestive tract, but make no mistake—there's an intimate connection between the two:

- Studies have found that more than half of all acne sufferers have alterations in gut flora, which affects their skin and bloats them, too.
- Societies that eat a more indigenous diet with little or no processed or sugary foods have very few digestive problems and virtually no acne.
- Rosacea has been linked to inflammation and bacterial imbalance in the gut, and it's one of the most common skin conditions I see in my bloated patients.

Your skin is like the outer aspect of your intestines: everything you eat eventually shows up on it, and, like bloating, skin reactions can be a sign of an unhappy gut. In addition to causing bloating, food allergies and food intolerances can also lead to dark circles under your eyes, blemishes, rashes, and a puffy, swollen appearance. My patients who have inflamed intestines frequently also have red, inflamed skin, and as their gut heals, their skin usually does, too.

Likewise, your intestines can be thought of as the innermost layer of your skin, since much of what you put on your skin eventually gets absorbed. Chemicals like sodium lauryl sulfate are common ingredients in cleansing products because they create a thick lather, but they're also easily absorbed through the skin, irritating it and stripping away essential oils and moisture. Harsh chemicals may make your skin more permeable to penetration by surface bacteria, viruses, and other chemicals that can gain access to your intestines and lead to inflammation and bloating.

GI Beauty Boosters

Your digestive system literally feeds your skin and hair, and there are two main mechanisms for how healthy insides can help make your outside healthy, too. The first is getting sufficient nutrients, both by eating them and by making sure your intestines are absorbing them properly, too. The second is maintaining bacterial balance and avoiding dysbiosis.

The Glow of Good Nutrition

If you have glowing skin and lustrous tresses, you may have been lucky in the gene pool, but you probably eat lots of fruits and vegetables, too. Nutritionally empty foods like most breakfast cereals and bread are fortified or enriched with minerals and vitamins, so you may think you're eating a healthy diet based on the ingredients list. But enriched food is a poor imitation of nutrient-rich food that naturally has the good stuff in it, or what I like to call food from the ground: foods like fruits, vegetables, legumes, nuts, and seeds. Ideally, you should be eating a rainbow of deeply pigmented foods. The different colors indicate the presence of different nutrients, and you need to eat a wide variety to make sure you're getting as many as possible. Green fruit like avocados and grapes provides nourishing B-complex vitamins, while oranges are rich in vitamin C, which helps reduce free-radical damage caused by sun exposure. The best way to make sure your skin and hair are getting lots of these nutrients is to eat foods that contain them. It's hard to fake this particular glow with a cream, just as taking a supplement or vitamin won't cure your bloating if you're eating an unhealthy diet.

You don't have to be a vegetarian to glow. Linda Petursdottir is an integrative nutritionist I work with who most definitely has inner and outer radiance. Here's how she describes her diet:

> *I am not a strict vegetarian or vegan but rather a flexetarian. My diet is mostly vegetarian with lots of veggies, fruit, beans, nuts, seeds and some grains, but I do eat fish and eggs and the occasional organic free-range poultry and, rarely, buffalo or Icelandic lamb. I would say I am 95% gluten- and dairy-free, but I do have a weakness for cheese.*

Eating in a way that's optimal for inner and outer health doesn't mean adhering to any particular dietary label, as long as you're eating nutrient-rich food and avoiding the unhealthy stuff. I know strict vegans who eat way too much sugar and processed foods and who are bloated with bad skin and thinning hair, and carnivores who also love veggies who look and feel amazing. It's not about applying labels or being "good" 100 percent of the time. It's about nourishing yourself from the inside out.

The Advantages of Absorption

If you've read some of the previous chapters, you know that dietary choices alone don't always dictate how nourished you are. You may be eating a very healthy diet but just not absorbing things properly. Acid-blocking drugs prescribed for reflux can decrease the absorption of nutrients, including fat-soluble vitamins important for healthy skin. The change in pH can also render digestive enzymes less effective, so you may have suboptimal digestion of protein and fat, causing lackluster skin and hair.

Gastrointestinal conditions like celiac disease and Crohn's can significantly alter absorption, and there's no question that in addition to bloating, they can also be accompanied by skin problems and hair loss. Almost 25 percent of people with celiac disease have a rash called dermatitis herpetiformis (DH). Both the rash and hair loss, which is an even more common complaint, usually respond dramatically to a gluten-free diet. Many of my patients who don't have celiac disease but who are gluten intolerant also have hair loss that improves after going off gluten.

Crohn's disease and ulcerative colitis can cause ulcers and nodules on the skin (pyoderma gangrenosum and erythema nodosum), and treating the inflammation in the gut also clears up the skin lesions, suggesting a direct relationship between the two. It's important to keep in mind that hair loss and acne in inflammatory conditions can also be caused by the medications we use to treat inflammation, particularly steroids and antibiotics—both major causes of bloating and key medications to try and avoid if you're suffering from blemished skin and thinning hair.

Regular alcohol consumption can take a serious toll on you, both inside and out. In addition to its bloating effects, alcohol dehydrates your skin, deprives it of vital nutrients and vitamins, and can trigger skin conditions like rosacea. Over time, this can have more permanent effects on your skin. Low iron levels from excessive alcohol may also cause hair loss.

The Bloom of Bacterial Balance

Bacterial imbalance, known as dysbiosis (see Chapter 6, "Trouble in the Microbiome?"), is one of the most pervasive causes of bloating and has an extremely detrimental effect on the microbiome, the microscopic environment of flora and fauna in our bodies. A nutrient-poor diet, frequent antibiotics, acid-suppressing drugs that alter the stomach's pH, infections, parasites, hormone therapy, steroids, and a host of other factors can lead to overgrowth of pathogenic or harmful bacteria and diminished numbers of essential good bacteria in the gut. But this imbalance also shows up on the skin and scalp, where it can profoundly affect your appearance. If you've taken lots of antibiotics or steroids, you may also have yeast overgrowth, which causes folliculitis, leading to hair loss and a red, scaly appearance of the scalp.

Antibiotics are a common treatment for acne and rosacea, but they're a shortsighted fix, since in the long run they can worsen those same skin conditions because of the development of dysbiosis, and also cause terrible bloating.

Dysbiosis is associated with a condition called leaky gut syndrome (see Chapter 14, "Could Your Gut Be Leaking?"), a state of increased permeability of the intestinal membranes strongly associated with bloating. Partially digested food, viruses, bacteria, and toxins normally excreted in the stool instead find their way through the intestinal membrane, where they can enter the bloodstream and trigger responses from different organs. Theories about what causes skin conditions like acne and rosacea include movement of toxins through the wall of the gut that then cause inflammation in the skin. Dysbiosis and leaky gut also prevent proper absorption of nutrients, which can bloat you and affect your appearance.

Identifying the cause of your bacterial imbalance and remediating it is an essential step in improving both your bloating and any associated skin or scalp conditions. You need healthy amounts of essential bacteria both in your GI tract and on your skin in order for them to function well. I recommend avoiding antibiotics unless absolutely necessary, since they wipe out healthy colonies of bacteria in the gut. Avoiding antibacterial soap that washes away healthy bacteria on the skin is just as essential.

What About Cleansing and Detoxification?

Can cleansing and detoxification lead to improvements in both your bloating and your appearance? Some people rave about the cleansed, glowing feeling they have after a colonic, while others feel dried out and dizzy. Colonic irrigation, hydrotherapy, or colonics refer to the practice of placing a tube into the rectum attached to special equipment through which large amounts of water, sometimes mixed with herbs or other substances, are pumped into the colon to remove waste matter. There is the possibility of minor complications such as infection from improperly cleaned equipment, dehydration, cramps and pain during the procedure, and electrolyte imbalances. Fortunately, more serious complications like heart failure from over-absorption of water and fatal perforation of the colon are extremely rare.

From my point of view, there are two drawbacks to colonics. The first is the potential disruption of the colon's unique and delicate bacterial environment when liquid is pumped in under high pressure. Although many practitioners of colonic irrigation claim that removing encrusted fecal matter in the colon actually enhances the growth of essential bacteria, the procedure can also indiscriminately wash away both good and bad species of bacteria, and taking a probiotic doesn't come close to replacing the essential flora that may be lost. The second drawback is the potential for dependency and colonic inertia (decreased motility) in people who undergo frequent colonics. The colon eventually realizes that much of its job is being done for it and may become less active in terms of contractility, leading to greater dependency on regular colonics for elimination.

Part of the popularity of colonics is that people feel really good when their colons are empty, and colonics are really good at emptying the colon. But the colon doesn't need much help eliminating waste matter when we're doing what we're supposed to be doing: eating a high-fiber, plant-based diet; avoiding processed food and sugar; drinking lots of water; and getting regular vigorous exercise. That will keep your bowels moving like clockwork and give you an all-over glow. For those who are wedded to the idea of a more drastic cleaning out, a two- or three-day green juice fast along with a couple of tablespoons of ground psyllium husk daily can give you pretty similar results, without disturbing your gut bacteria.

The Bottom Line

Ultimately, the less toxic your lifestyle, the less need you'll have for detoxification. While I'm not recommending that you go back to the cave or forgo technology, when it comes to healthy intestines and skin, it's hard to improve on what nature provides. When you kill off large amounts of essential gut bacteria with antibiotics, they can't simply be replaced with an off-the-shelf product. Likewise, important skin bacteria and its natural moisture and oils that are washed away by harsh chemicals can't be restored with manufactured products. And no amount of vitamins or supplements can take the place of a balanced, nutrient-rich diet.

My 10-Day Gutbliss Plan (see Chapter 23) is a great way to banish bloat and improve the health of your skin and hair at the same time. Many of the tips I describe below are an integral part of the plan.

Gutbliss Spa: Beauty Recipes for Skin and Hair

I've been reading nutrition labels on items at the grocery store for many years, but after my daughter was born I started paying more attention to the ingredients labels on personal care products such as shampoo and lotion that I was using on both her and myself. I was shocked when I started

Gutbliss Solutions for Eating Your Way to a More Beautiful You

- **Eat dark green vegetables.** Arguably they're the single best food group for promoting healthy skin. No other food group can match the water content and pound-for-pound nutrient density of dark green vegetables and their high vitamin C content helps the body make skin-firming collagen. I recommend shooting for one head of romaine lettuce or three stalks of kale every day.

- **Eat foods rich in omega-3 fatty acids and flavonoids.** Both groups of nutrients are strongly associated with healthy blood vessels, which are essential for maintaining optimal blood flow to and from your skin cells. Healthy foods that are naturally rich in omega-3 fatty acids include: dark green leafy vegetables, raw walnuts, wild salmon, flax seeds, and free-range eggs. Healthy foods that are naturally rich in flavonoids include: lettuce, cherries, citrus, cabbage, kale, spinach, Goji berries, asparagus, lima beans, and raw cacao.

- **Eat foods rich in vitamin A, carotenoids, and healthy fats.** Vitamin A is one of the most important micronutrients for healthy skin, since it's needed to maintain the integrity and function of your skin cells. If your overall health is good and you regularly eat foods that are abundant in healthy fats, then chances are that your body is effectively synthesizing vitamin A from carotenoids found in dark green, yellow, and orange vegetables such as spinach, carrots, and sweet potatoes.

- **Cut down on sugar.** Prevent dysbiosis and yeast overgrowth in your gut and on your skin by keeping sweet treats that yeast thrive on to a minimum. Sugary foods also promote insulin release, and high circulating insulin levels are associated with inflammation throughout the body, including your GI tract and your skin.

- **Don't add salt.** Adding salt to food causes water retention, making you bloated and puffy all over, especially in your face. Food manufacturers often add salt to packaged food to preserve its shelf life, so even if you put away the salt shaker, you still need to read labels to keep your salt intake in check. Aim for 1,000 milligrams or less per day.

- **Avoid gluten.** The gluten-containing grains of today are a modified version of what our ancestors ate and have been associated with lots of different symptoms, including bloating, rashes, and hair loss. Even if you don't have celiac disease, you may be gluten intolerant and not even know it. A six-week trial of a gluten-free diet that excludes wheat, rye, and barley may do wonders for blemished skin, thinning hair, and bloating.
- **Be a teetotaler.** Alcohol is metabolized to acetaldehyde, a cousin of formaldehyde and a substance that's toxic to practically every organ system. And did I mention it can cause bloating and blotchy skin, make your hair fall out, and age you?
- **Limit dairy.** Although the party line from most dermatologists is that acne isn't related to diet, many studies show an increase in acne incidence and severity in people who consume lots of dairy. It's also a major cause of bloating, since more than half the world's population is lactose intolerant.
- **Hydrate.** It seems obvious, but if you're not measuring how much water you're drinking, chances are you're not drinking enough. Your thirst mechanism doesn't kick in until you're already pretty dehydrated, and then it's hard to catch up. Water helps to move the products of digestion through the colon, avoiding backup, which can lead to toxins leaching into your blood supply and traveling to the rest of your body, including your skin. Drinking lots of water also helps you get rid of toxins through your body's largest organ of elimination—your skin. Be sure to avoid caffeine and soda, which can actually dehydrate you.

researching the side effects of many of the chemical ingredients, and I was struck by the similarities between the food industry and personal products industry: aggressive marketing of long-shelf-life products that are cheap to manufacture and use lots of inexpensive chemicals and fillers. I eventually stopped buying these products and started whipping up my own at home. I continue to be amazed at the superior quality of these homemade products in terms of their ability to exfoliate and moisturize, and they smell and feel terrific. Over the years my daughter and I have

Gutbliss Solutions for How to Be a Product Detective

- **Don't use dirty products.** If you use "dirty" products full of chemicals on your body, you're destroying the delicate ecosystem on your skin that's essential for its health. Most of what tries to pass itself off as science, encouraging you to buy fancy products with lots of ingredients you've never heard of, is really just marketing—the same kind that claims a candy bar with fake protein is health food. Michael Pollan's famous food rule #2 also applies to the skin: *Don't put anything on your skin with more than five ingredients, or ingredients you can't pronounce.*
- **Use edible products.** This may sound a little odd, but remember that your skin is a porous membrane: it absorbs ("eats") what you put on it, which ends up inside you. Apply the same philosophy to your skin and hair care that you follow in the kitchen: use high-quality, simple ingredients straight from nature, not from the lab. Raw honey, papaya, oatmeal, and coconut oil will serve you just as well in the bathroom as they do in the kitchen. Check out my amazing edible skin and hair-care recipes in this chapter.

created many wonderful recipes for skin and hair care that are literally good enough to eat. Below are some of our favorite beauty recipes.

Simple Facial Wash

2 tablespoons raw honey

❋ Moisten your face and hands with water and gently rub the honey all over your face in a circular motion for 1 minute. Wash off with lukewarm water and a clean, wet washcloth. This facial wash can be used daily. Honey has an optimal pH that helps to balance the skin, and is rich in minerals and moisture, making it a perfect base for facial recipes.

Gutbliss Solutions for a Beautiful Lifestyle

- **Live inside out.** Nourish your microbiome by creating the most hospitable environment for good bacteria to flourish, not just in your gut but also on your skin and scalp. That means avoiding unnecessary antibiotics, harsh chemicals, and other drugs that can kill off essential bacteria, and eating lots of high-fiber foods, such as leafy greens, that encourage the growth of beneficial species. Adding good bacteria to your microbiome can help, too. Probiotics are live strains of bacteria that can be taken in a pill, powder, or liquid form. I usually recommend a ninety-day course of a robust probiotic containing large amounts of helpful bacteria like *Lactobacillus* and *Bifidobacterium*. Although there can be some worsening of bloating initially, you should notice improvement in both your GI symptoms and your skin after about a month.

- **Don't be too clean.** Lathering your skin and hair every day strips away the essential oils and moisture that are created by your body for your specific pH. They definitely can't be replaced with some department store version, even the super expensive kind. Most of the time we're really not that dirty, and a quick rinse with just water will do. Get in and out of the shower in less than five minutes and use lukewarm rather than hot water to avoid drying out your skin.

- **Get a showerhead filter.** A charcoal filter in your showerhead can help to remove chlorine and other chemicals in water than can thin and dry out your hair.

- **Move.** Exercise is one of the best ways to improve your internal and external appearance. Get sweaty as often as you can, ideally at least three times a week. Running, brisk walking, yoga, karate, soccer, dancing, tennis, boot camp, swimming—it's all good. Exercise improves digestion and the rhythmic contractions of your GI system called peristalsis, which help to reduce bloating. It also increases blood flow to the skin, which is how skin gets its nutrients. Plus, it releases feel-good endorphins that give you a great glow.

Oily Skin Facial Scrub

2 tablespoons raw honey

1 teaspoon oatmeal

½ teaspoon cornmeal

½ teaspoon lemon juice

❊ Moisten your face and hands with water and mix all the ingredients in the palms of your hands. Gently rub the paste all over your face in a circular motion for 1 minute. The cornmeal and lemon juice are great natural exfoliants, but if you apply too much pressure or scrub too hard, you can irritate your skin. Wash off with lukewarm water and a clean wet washcloth. This facial scrub can be used once a week. Make a larger batch to use on the rest of your body.

Dry Skin Facial Scrub

2 tablespoons raw honey

2 tablespoons crushed fresh ripe papaya (skin and seeds removed)

1 teaspoon oatmeal

❊ Moisten your face and hands with water and mix all of the ingredients in the palms of your hands. Gently rub the paste all over your face and neck in a circular motion. Massage for 1 to 2 minutes. Wash off with lukewarm water and a clean wet washcloth. This facial scrub can be used once a week. Make a larger batch to use on the rest of your body.

Coconut Oil Exfoliating/Moisturizing Body Scrub

4 tablespoons raw honey

2 tablespoons coconut oil

1 tablespoon cornmeal

❊ Moisten your body and hands with water and mix all of the ingredients in the palms of your hands. Gently rub the paste all over your body, paying special attention to any rough patches of skin. Wash off with lukewarm water and a clean wet washcloth. This body scrub can be used daily.

Warm Brown Sugar Exfoliating/ Moisturizing Body Scrub

3 tablespoons coconut oil

2 tablespoons brown sugar

2 tablespoons raw honey

1 tablespoon vanilla essence

❖ In a small pan, combine all of the ingredients and heat gently until the coconut oil is completely liquid and the brown sugar has dissolved. Mix well. Allow the paste to cool to a comfortable temperature. Then gently massage it all over your body. Wash it off with lukewarm water and a clean wet washcloth. This body scrub can be used daily.

Vanilla Moisturizing Lotion

2 tablespoons coconut oil

1 tablespoon jojoba oil

½ teaspoon vanilla essence

❖ Mix all of the ingredients well in the palms of your hands or in a small bowl and apply liberally all over your body. This moisturizing lotion can be used daily.

Citrus Moisturizing Lotion

2 tablespoons coconut oil

1 tablespoon jojoba oil

½ teaspoon grated orange or lemon zest

❖ Mix all of the ingredients well in the palms of your hands or in a small bowl and apply liberally all over your body. This moisturizing lotion can be used daily.

Moisturizing Hair Mask for Dry/Damaged Hair

2 tablespoons coconut oil

1 tablespoon olive oil

1 ripe avocado

❋ In a small bowl, combine all of the ingredients and mix well to form a paste. Apply the paste to wet hair, working it through from the roots to the ends. Wrap the hair in a warm towel or plastic wrap and leave the paste in for 30 minutes. Rinse well with lukewarm water. Do not shampoo or condition the hair afterward. Use once a month.

Rinse for Oily Hair

1 cup apple cider vinegar

1 cup water

❋ In a bowl, combine the apple cider vinegar and water. Apply to wet hair, working it through from the roots to the ends and massaging it into the scalp. Leave in for 5 minutes and then rinse with water. Do not shampoo or condition the hair afterward. Use once a month. NOTE: This formulation will strip color if your hair is colored with hair dye or henna.

I spend a fair amount of time in people's digestive tracts. It's unusual to see great insides and a bad outside, and vice versa, especially after age thirty, when we stop having the faces and bodies we're born with and start having the ones that reflect how we're living. Benjamin Franklin said, "While we may not be able to control all that happens to us, we can control what happens inside us." I don't think he was referring to the GI tract, but it certainly applies. I hope this chapter will motivate you to find your glow from the inside out, while banishing your bloat at the same time.

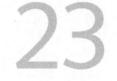

Ten Days to Gutbliss

I'M AN ADVOCATE OF DO-IT-YOURSELF MEDICINE. I FERVENTLY BELIEVE that most of us have the ability to heal what ails us through paying close attention to the cues our body gives us and making the necessary adjustments to our diet and lifestyle. More and more evidence points to what we eat and how we live, rather than genetics, as the underlying causes behind cancer, heart disease, diabetes, high blood pressure, stroke, and, of course, digestive ailments.

Hippocrates said that *all disease begins in the gut*—and he was right. A clogged, unhealthy digestive system doesn't just bloat you; it weighs you down in so many other ways, affecting your mood, energy level, libido, and overall sense of well-being. Autoimmune diseases, inflammation, allergies, and even cancer often start in the GI tract, when toxins gain access to the bloodstream through a damaged intestinal lining, poisoning the rest of the body.

In the previous chapters, we looked at ways you can learn to read your digestive road map, making changes along the route to improved health and well-being. In fact, with every new day, you have a new opportunity to take control of your body, your bloating, and your life. My 10-Day Gutbliss Plan will show you how.

The 10-Day Gutbliss Plan isn't a diet. It's a commitment to making a few simple but significant changes for a relatively short period of time that will help you banish bloat, flush toxins, and dump your digestive baggage—the healthy way. It has helped thousands of women tighten their tummies and end their discomfort, as well as boost their energy and mood by optimizing levels of serotonin, the feel-good hormone located in the gut.

Food as Medicine, Food as Bliss

"What should I eat?" is the question I'm asked the most by patients. It's also the question I wrestle with the most myself. I don't endorse any particular way to eat, other than increasing the things that are good for you and decreasing those that aren't, cooking most of your food yourself, as well as trying to be an ethical consumer. Some days, fruits, vegetables, beans, healthy grains, and a little animal protein seem right; on others, a gluten-free vegan diet makes me feel best. I've learned to stay flexible and listen to what my body wants and also not to drive myself crazy in search of an idealized notion of the perfect diet. I designed my plan to be adjustable enough to fit your busy life and your individual needs. For those of you who like a more structured approach, My Gutbliss 10-Day Meal Plan on page 238 takes you step by step through what ten days of my own blissful eating looks like. And have fun in the kitchen trying out the Gutbliss Recipes starting on page 247!

Gutbliss Guidelines

Food is medicine for your body. But keeping up with the latest nutritional science can feel like a full-time job, and eating is also about simple, beautiful ingredients and pleasure. That's why my Gutbliss Plan focuses on bliss, not perfection. Below are some general guidelines to keep in mind.

STOP COUNTING, START ENJOYING

My plan doesn't involve counting calories or calculating net carbs. Food is much more than just its constituent parts. Forget about how many grams of protein something has and think about whether the food you're eating is helping you or harming you, whether it's just filler that's not making a difference either way, or whether it's even food at all.

Simply fill your plate with food that's as close to its natural state as possible: potatoes instead of potato chips, apples instead of applesauce. Avoid packaged products with long ingredients lists and extended shelf lives, and beware of marketing masquerading as science. Remember my basic definition of food that doesn't require a calculator or advanced degree to figure out: *something that nourishes you.* I recommend that you strive to eat the absolute best food you can get your hands on, every day, because although it won't be perfect, it really is your best medicine.

LISTEN TO YOUR BODY

The gastrointestinal tract has an amazing capacity to recover and heal, and it wants to be healthy. The bloating you experience is its way of communicating with you, giving you critical feedback that something isn't right and asking you to make a change. What you eat and how you live have a much greater impact on your digestive health than anything else, and this is exactly what we'll be focusing on with the plan.

The Gutbliss Plan is based on the initiatives I've found to be the most effective for bloating and digestive distress in my patients. Some are things you might already be doing, but I encourage you to follow all the steps of the plan, as you'll see the best results if you do them together. It's incredibly rewarding to have patients tell me how much better they feel after implementing these changes, and I'm excited to share this program with you.

EAT REAL FOOD

While you're on the plan, there are a few foods you'll need to *eliminate* completely, others I'll ask you to *limit*, and some I'll recommend you go out of your way to *include* on a daily basis. There'll still be plenty to eat and lots of opportunity to enjoy a nice meal at a restaurant or with friends.

What can you eat on the plan? Real food, and plenty of it—especially nutrient-dense vegetables, fruits, nuts, seeds, and some whole grains. High-quality animal protein is allowed but not required.

What should you avoid? Processed foods, chemicals in food, and foods that are notorious for producing bloating.

At the end of the ten-day period, you can continue all of the changes, or just the ones that made the most difference for you. They all lead to better health. What about life after that? I recommend the 80 percent rule: try to stick to the principles behind the plan 80 percent of the time. That's enough to maintain the digestive advantage you've created, while also allowing you to live in the real world.

As part of your new blissful lifestyle, dip into Chapter 22 for Gutbliss Spa recipes for skin and hair care that are literally good enough to eat. Other lifestyle recommendations in the plan involve nourishing mind-body practices and any exercise that helps you sweat out your toxins. We'll even talk about how to "turn around and take a look" as part of achieving stool nirvana—something few diet gurus discuss but which is a crucial part of banishing your bloat. Since you're not under my care, I can't give you specific medical advice, but I'll share some important information about medications that could be contributing to your bloat and a few products that might improve it.

The 10-Day Gutbliss Plan

The 10-Day Gutbliss Plan removes the six foods I've identified as the most problematic for bloating and digestive upset. It can be hard to assess cause and effect when you eat something all the time and you're bloated all the time, too. Is it just coincidence, or could there be a connection? Ten days might not be adequate time for your symptoms to completely resolve, but it should be enough time for you to notice real improvement. At the end of the ten-day period, you can continue to permanently exclude all the foods on the list, or reintroduce one item a week to see which ones give you the most trouble and which ones you can tolerate. For most of my patients, eliminating these six foods leads to a dramatic improvement in their bloating, even if they're dealing with additional factors, such as a poorly functioning thyroid gland or diverticulosis.

THE BIG SIX: FOODS TO ELIMINATE

The Big Six foods you'll be eliminating are easy to remember because they spell the words SAD GAS. These are foods you should completely avoid while you're on the plan:

Soy
Artificial sweeteners
Dairy
Gluten
Alcohol
Sugar

Let's look at each in more detail.

Soy

Eliminate processed soy products, including soy milk, tofu, soy yogurt, and soy cheeses. Avoid products containing soy protein isolate, a common filler in packaged food.

Processed soy can have estrogen-like effects that contribute to bloating and weight gain.

Artificial Sweeteners

Eliminate all low-calorie and zero-calorie sweeteners, including sugar alcohols such as sorbitol, mannitol, erythritol, and xylitol. Avoid aspartame, saccharin, and sucralose, too. Also eliminate diet sodas and diet drinks and any foods sweetened with artificial sweeteners.

Incomplete absorption of artificial sweeteners in the small intestine leads to fermentation by colonic bacteria, causing lots of gas and bloating.

Dairy

Eliminate dairy, including yogurt, cheese, milk, butter, buttermilk, cream, whey products, and ice cream. Acceptable dairy alternatives include almond milk, coconut milk, rice milk, and hemp milk. Make sure to get the unsweetened and unflavored kind.

More than half the world is lactose intolerant, and that may include you. Classic symptoms are gas, bloating, and abdominal cramps. Some commercial dairy cows are treated with hormones that have estrogen-like effects that may worsen bloating.

Gluten

Eliminate wheat, rye, and barley, all of which contain gluten. Now, this part is really important: try not to simply swap all your gluten-containing foods for gluten-free versions, since what you'll be doing is swapping one processed carbohydrate for another. Instead, use this as an opportunity to explore other healthy grains such as brown rice, amaranth, and millet, as well as quinoa (which is actually a seed).

Gluten-free living isn't just a fad. Almost 1 percent of the population in the United States has celiac disease, and millions more suffer from gluten intolerance. The small intestine isn't designed to digest processed gluten-containing grains, and bloating is one of the most common reactions.

Alcohol

Eliminate alcohol of all kinds, including beer, wine, champagne, gin, vodka, tequila, rum, et cetera. Avoid nonalcoholic beer because it's made from the same ingredients as regular beer.

Alcohol bloats you in a number of ways: it's made from fermented grains that can be irritating to the small intestine; it damages the lining of the stomach, causing inflammation; it can impair release of digestive enzymes from the pancreas; it adds pounds to your waistline by slowing the body's fat-burning ability; it dehydrates you, causing fluid retention and puffiness.

Sugar

Eliminate foods with any added sugars. Look out for hidden sugars in ingredients lists, including glucose, fructose, maltose, dextrose, and corn syrup. Avoid naturally occurring sweeteners like honey, agave, maple syrup, and stevia, also. Do not drink soda, fruit juices, or other beverages containing any of these sweeteners. Naturally occurring sugar and fructose in fruits and vegetables is fine.

Sugar doesn't bring much to the table in terms of nutritional value, but it can bring a lot of bloat. It's the preferred food for gas-producing bacteria and undesirable yeast species like candida and can lead to bacterial imbalance called dysbiosis, a major cause of bloating. It also leads to stubborn belly fat by flooding your system with insulin. Fructose is a common sweetener in soda and processed foods, but 30 percent of the population has fructose malabsorption, resulting in fermentation by colonic bacteria and lots of gas.

FOODS TO LIMIT

Some of these foods are actually good for you but, nonetheless, can cause a lot of bloating. Others aren't so healthy but are well tolerated in small amounts if you feel like you can't give them up altogether.

Beans, Broccoli, and Cabbage

These foods are notorious for causing bloating, but they have lots of health benefits, so I never recommend cutting them out altogether, although smaller servings and a little Beano can go a long way. If you tolerate them or don't mind the gas, there's no need to limit them at all.

Carbonated Beverages

Carbonated beverages such as seltzer water can bloat you because of the carbon dioxide bubbles, which fill you with gas. They sometimes have added salt, too. While you're on the plan, I recommend choosing flat water over fizzy.

Caffeine

Caffeine works as a laxative for some people, but its stimulant effect can also cause cramping and bloating. While you're on the plan, limit your caffeine intake to no more than one small cup of coffee or tea daily.

Fatty Foods

You know they can pack on the pounds, but they also slow movement through the gastrointestinal tract because they're harder to digest, making you feel full and bloated. Avoid heavy meals, fried foods, and rich sauces while you're on the plan.

Meat

If you're going to eat animal protein (beef, poultry, wild game, lamb, pork, et cetera) while you're on the plan, it should be organic and grass-fed. The chemicals, hormones, and antibiotics in a lot of factory-farmed meats and poultry disrupt your microbiome and can contribute to estrogen dominance. Because meat has a higher fat content, it's harder to digest and can slow down your GI transit time, so limit animal protein to one meal a day or none at all if you can do without it.

Processed Foods

These foods usually contain sugar, artificial sweeteners, dairy, gluten, or soy—but even those that don't should be avoided. Eat food that's as close to its natural state as possible: for example, apples instead of applesauce. Avoid packaged products with long ingredients lists and lengthy expiration dates, and beware of marketing masquerading as science.

Salt

Salt can be difficult to avoid because it's added to most prepared and packaged foods and is also used as a preservative. While you're on the plan, don't add salt to your food and limit total daily consumption to no more than 1,000 milligrams.

FOODS TO INCLUDE

Some foods are particularly helpful when it comes to banishing bloat and healing the GI tract because they encourage the growth of healthy bacteria, provide digestive enzymes, or create bulk, which aids elimination. Aim to consume 50 percent of your food every day in its natural, raw state to maximize the effectiveness of the digestive enzymes that are present in the food. That way, your GI tract won't have to work as hard to digest it. That means lots of fresh fruit, salads, nuts, and seeds. Eat the healthiest and best-quality food you can get your hands on every day. It really is your best medicine!

Greens

Greens are the least consumed food in the standard American diet, yet they're the most essential for inner and outer health. They come the closest of any food to meeting our ideal nutritional requirements. It probably wouldn't surprise you to know that romaine lettuce has more fiber than sirloin, but you may not know that calorie for calorie, it has double the protein, ten times the amount of iron, and a hundred times more calcium. If you asked me to recommend the one thing that would have the biggest impact on your bloating and overall digestive health, it would be to eat as many leafy green vegetables as you can.

If you want to encourage the growth of good bacteria, heal inflammation, improve motility, crowd out parasites, eliminate yeast, get rid of belly fat, dissolve gallstones, balance your pH, quiet down your irritable bowel syndrome (IBS), prevent diverticulosis, cut your risk of colon cancer in half, boost your energy, lose weight, banish your bloat, and really glow, then the single most important thing you need to do is eat greens every single day. There's a lot to choose from: kale, spinach, chard, collards, parsley, turnip greens, mustard greens, dandelion greens, beet greens, arugula, broccoli, bok choy, and all kinds of lettuce. And a lot of ways to fix them: steamed, sautéed, stir-fried, boiled, roasted, raw, in salads, in smoothies, or on their own. However you eat them, leafy greens are the embodiment of food as medicine. You don't have to like them; you just have to eat them. If you do nothing else, commit to eating leafy greens every day for the next ten days and I promise you, amazing things will start to happen inside and out.

High-Fiber Foods

High-fiber foods keep your digestive pipes clean, but too much fiber at one time can actually clog them, so you may need to spread your fiber out in small increments throughout the day, or start with small servings and gradually increase them. You should be eating plant-based fiber from fruits and vegetables at every meal. Processed fiber from cereals, muffins, and other baked goods is far less helpful with bloating and bowel movements.

Papaya and Pineapple

These luscious fruits contain papain and bromelain, respectively, which are potent protease enzymes that break down protein and can even be used as meat tenderizers. Try to include a fresh serving of either of these two fruits daily if they're in season—not too hard to do, seeing as they are colorful, sweet treats!

Colored Produce

Brightly colored produce—crimson strawberries, bright orange bell peppers, sunny yellow lemons, deep green spinach—contain essential vitamins and minerals needed to enhance digestion and keep your microbiome healthy. Eating a veritable rainbow of deeply pigmented fruits and vegetables will not only keep the bloat away, it will repair nutrient deficiencies you didn't even know you had, boost your mood, and dramatically improve the appearance of your skin.

Water, Water, Water, and More Water

Drinking two liters of fresh, still, tap, purified, or spring water daily is one of the most important aspects of the plan and a must to keep your digestive pipes unclogged and bloat-free.

Fresh Vegetable Juice

Fresh veggie juice is full of nutrients. While it's not a substitute for eating vegetables because the juicing process removes the fiber, it's a great addition to all the other things you're doing on the plan and provides an additional beverage option. Make sure the kind you're drinking is fresh, preferably made just before drinking or within twenty-four hours of consuming. Avoid packaged, premade vegetable juices that have a lot of sugar and may be pasteurized to extend their shelf life.

Fennel Tea

This tea is a great bloat buster. Fennel is a member of the carrot and parsley family and has a long history of medicinal use. Fennel helps to relax your digestive tract and eliminate gas and also aids digestion by enhancing production of gastric juices. Use whole fennel seeds boiled in water to make the tea; then strain the tea to remove the seeds before drinking.

My Magic Smoothie

I love my Magic Smoothie. It's full of live food and bloat-busting fiber and is a great way to start the day. It's an outstanding alternative to breakfast cereal that's been sitting in a box for months or pancakes or muffins that are broken down into pure sugar that results in excess gas production, weight gain, and inflammation. I recommend having this smoothie every day while you're on the plan, for breakfast in the morning or as a snack later in the day. Here's the recipe:

In a blender, combine:

1 sliced ripe banana

2 cups mixed berries

1 cup raw spinach, kale, collards, or chard, washed (central stem removed for the kale/collards/chard)

1 tablespoon ground psyllium husk

1 tablespoon ground flax seed

1 cup crushed ice

1 cup almond milk, coconut milk, or coconut water.

❊ Blend well and drink immediately. Makes 2 large servings.

How to Eat

When it comes to bloating, *how* you eat can be as important as *what* you eat, particularly if you're swallowing large amounts of air with your food or you're consuming the majority of your calories at night.

REDUCE AIR SWALLOWING

This is a major source of bloating that you can easily reduce by drinking and eating separately, not at the same time. Also, chew each bite of food at least twenty times before swallowing. Not only will you swallow less air, but also more salivary enzymes will be released, making it easier for your body to digest the food. Try not to talk while eating. Finally, avoid chewing gum and sucking on hard candy or mints.

GIVE YOUR TUMMY A BEDTIME

Gastric emptying slows down considerably once the sun sets. Make sure that's not when you're dumping in the majority of your calories, or you'll find yourself bloated and uncomfortable at night. You shouldn't be eating beyond an hour after sunset while you're on the plan.

Shift your calorie consumption to the times when you need them the most and when your digestive tract is the most active: in the morning and daytime. I recommend eating breakfast like a queen, lunch like a princess, and dinner like a pauper.

Supplements

Philosophically, I believe you can get all the nutrients you need from food, so I don't recommend taking additional vitamins or supplements unless you have a specific deficiency that's been identified. But even people who eat a high-fiber diet can benefit from a fiber supplement, and given the multiple factors that lead to bacterial imbalance, a robust probiotic is often helpful.

PSYLLIUM

Think of psyllium as a broom that sweeps debris out of your colon and keeps the products of digestion moving through efficiently. Even if you follow a high-fiber diet, you can still benefit from the additional fiber in psyllium.

While you're on the plan, take one tablespoon of psyllium twice daily mixed in a large glass of water and immediately followed by an additional glass of water. You can add a splash of unsweetened juice for flavor or use a flavored type of psyllium; just make sure it doesn't contain any artificial sweeteners. If you find that psyllium is making you more bloated, try reducing the dose to a twice-daily teaspoon instead of a tablespoon.

PROBIOTICS

Probiotics are supplements that contain large amounts of live bacteria. They can help repopulate the colon with essential species and restore balance if you've been taking antibiotics, acid suppressors, birth control pills, hormone replacement therapy, or steroids, or have a starchy, sugary diet that contributes to bacterial imbalance. Probiotics can help build and maintain a healthy digestive system by improving the barrier function of the intestinal lining and enhancing nutrient absorption.

While you're on the plan, take a daily robust probiotic, preferably one containing large amounts of *Bifidobacterium* and *Lactobacillus*.

Medications to Avoid

Although I believe in the concept of food as medicine, I also believe that there are times when both prescription and over-the-counter medications may be necessary. Unfortunately, many commonly prescribed drugs like the ones listed below are overprescribed and can lead to significant bloating and digestive upset, so try to avoid them whenever possible.

ANTIBIOTICS

There's no question that antibiotics can be lifesaving in the right setting, but they are often unnecessarily prescribed. Each dose of antibiotic kills off massive amounts of essential bacteria, contributing to dysbiosis and the overgrowth of bloat-causing yeast species. Avoid antibiotics unless you're seriously ill and the doctor doesn't think you'll get better without them. Minor infections will often heal on their own, particularly if you're enhancing your immune system with lots of fruits and vegetables. Remember, soup and rest do wonders for the common cold; antibiotics do nothing.

NONSTEROIDAL ANTI-INFLAMMATORY DRUGS

These medications, also known as NSAIDs, may help inflammation in your joints, but they can cause damage to the lining of the GI tract, leading to bloating and digestive distress. Avoid taking these medications whenever possible. If you have arthritis or chronic pain, ask your doctor whether a non-NSAID alternative might be an option.

ACID-SUPPRESSIVE MEDICATIONS

These include proton pump inhibitors, histamine blockers, and antacids, all of which decrease acid in the GI tract. The problem is that acid is the body's main defense against invading bacteria, and it provides the optimum pH for digestive enzymes and absorption of nutrients. Decreasing stomach acid is a major cause of bloating. Avoid any and all medications that interfere with stomach acid production. Instead, focus on ways to decrease heartburn naturally, by cutting back on caffeine, alcohol, fatty foods, large meals, and late-night eating.

HORMONES

The hormones in birth control pills and hormone replacement therapy can create a situation of estrogen dominance, which contributes to bloating. They can also disrupt the delicate balance of bacteria in the GI tract. Consider switching to a nonhormonal form of birth control, such as the copper IUD (intrauterine device) or condoms.

STEROIDS

Steroids are used to quiet inflammation in a number of different conditions, but they can lead to yeast overgrowth in the intestines and to severe dysbiosis and bloating. Even steroid creams applied to the skin can be absorbed in sufficient quantities to have these effects if they're used for long enough and in high enough concentrations. Avoid steroid preparations whenever possible.

The Gutbliss Life

There are lots of things you can do on a daily basis to help banish your bloat, from abdominal massage to yoga. Here are some of my favorites.

HAPPY ABS: ABDOMINAL SELF-MASSAGE

I recommend using a two- to five-pound dumbbell. Lie on your back and hold the weight in your right hand. Rest it on your abdomen and, applying gentle pressure, move it in a clockwise direction, making a large circle around your belly button. Try not to do this right after eating when your stomach may still be full. At night before bed or in the morning before breakfast is an ideal time.

SWEET BREATHING

Place one hand on your chest and the other on your abdomen. As you inhale slowly, your bottom hand should move up and out and your top hand and your shoulders should remain relatively quiet. As you exhale, your bottom hand should move back in. (If you're having trouble with this, place a five-pound bag of rice on your abdomen so that you have a physical sensation of where to place the breath.)

Now take a slow breath in your chest and notice how it produces tension in your neck, shoulders, stomach, and back. Now exhale, allowing all of the tension to leave your body. Notice how tension is associated with "chest" breathing and the relaxed feeling you have when you breathe diaphragmatically, that is, when the abdomen moves in and out and the upper body stays quiet.

- Inhale to a slow count of 4 (inflate the abdomen).
- Exhale to a slow count of 6 (deflate the abdomen).
- Modify to a count of 3 for inhalation and 5 for exhalation if necessary for comfort.

Regardless of the count, your focus should be on exhalation, which should be longer than inhalation. If at all possible, practice for twenty to thirty minutes twice a day to truly realize a change in how your body reacts to stress.

MOVE YOUR BODY!

How often and how vigorously you exercise will depend on your baseline level of activity, but I recommend that while you're on the plan you do at least thirty minutes of motion every day that's vigorous enough to make you sweat. This is key because when you sweat, you're also eliminating toxins through your largest organ—your skin. In addition to exercise, daily use of a steam room or sauna (if you don't have any medical contraindications) can help you eliminate toxins through your skin and will enhance the dietary and other lifestyle steps you're taking.

Having a massage on a regular basis is a luxury, but one that's definitely worth the expense, so while you're on the plan, think about saving the dollars you might once have spent on prepared foods, sweet treats, or gourmet coffee and put them toward a pair of magic hands. Studies have found massage beneficial for stress relief, anxiety, depression, boosting immunity, treating pain, improving stiffness, and even cancer therapy. Massage also has a hugely beneficial effect on the GI tract, particularly in people with IBS and chronic abdominal pain.

SKIN AND HAIR CARE RECIPES GOOD ENOUGH TO EAT

Check out Chapter 22, "Beauty and the Bloat," for my favorite edible recipes for lotions and potions you can easily make at home to help keep your hair and skin beautiful and free of unnecessary chemicals.

My Gutbliss 10-Day Meal Plan

I spend a lot of time giving people advice about what to eat, as well as ruminating on what works best for my own body, taste buds, and schedule. What's clear to me is that creating bliss in your gut isn't just about eliminating things like SAD GAS (see page 227) that can be a problem. It's also about making sure you include enough of the foods that provide the essential nutrients your digestive tract needs for optimal function.

I avoid SAD GAS about 80 percent of the time (except for artificial sweeteners, which I never use), and that gives me enough flexibility to eat out, experiment with new recipes, and indulge when I feel like it. Most of the food I eat on a daily basis is easy to prepare, great tasting, and nutrient-rich, and it makes me (and my GI tract) feel good after eating it. To accomplish that, I keep these five basic principles in mind when I'm planning my meals:

1. Encourage the growth of good bacteria with high-fiber prebiotic foods.
2. Obtain the necessary micronutrients from brightly colored fruits and vegetables.

3. Eat at least 50 percent of the food raw for added enzymes and more nutrients.
4. Eat animal protein no more than once a day, to make room for phyto-nutrients.
5. Batch-cook at the beginning of the week to have lots of options for lunches and dinners and use leftovers liberally.

Here's what a typical week of gutbliss looks like for me:

(B = breakfast; L = lunch; D = dinner; S = snack)

*NOTE: For recipes marked by an asterisk (*), please see the Gutbliss Recipes section in the Appendix.

Day 1

B: Dr. Chutkan's Magic Smoothie,* ½ grapefruit, and mint tea with lemon
L: Chopped kale salad with cabbage and Spicy Roasted Chickpeas* over brown rice
S: 1 orange, 1 apple, and a handful of raw almonds
D: Lemony Roasted Chicken,* roasted sweet potatoes and carrots, and sautéed string beans
S: Blackberries sprinkled with "crust" made from almond meal mixed with coconut oil and baked in the oven for 10 minutes

Day 2

B: Green Smoothie* and ½ grapefruit
L: Spicy Black Beans* over brown rice
S: 2 plums, 1 pear, and carrots and hummus
D: Lemony Roasted Chicken,* chopped kale salad, and brown rice
S: 1 orange, 1 apple, and mint tea with lemon

Day 3

B: Steel-Cut Oats with Berries and Flax Seeds,* 2 fried eggs, and freshly made green juice (kale, spinach, and green apple)

L: Flax seed crackers with hummus, 1 carrot, and 2 small apples

S: Handful of raw almonds and dried cranberries

D: Split Pea Soup/Dal* over brown rice with sautéed spinach

S: Frozen banana blended with almond milk, almonds, and unsweetened cocoa powder

Day 4

B: Dr. Chutkan's Magic Smoothie,* ½ grapefruit, and flax seed crackers with almond butter

L: Split Pea Soup/Dal* over brown rice

S: Sliced banana, strawberries, and gluten-free granola with almond milk

D: Noah's Asian Turkey Sliders,* Braised Baby Bok Choy,* and brown rice

S: Frozen banana blended with almond milk, almonds, and unsweetened cocoa powder

Day 5

B: Smoked salmon with scrambled eggs, plus a Green Smoothie*

L: Noah's Asian Turkey Sliders,* Braised Baby Bok Choy,* and brown rice

D: Rainbow Salad,* plus corn tortillas with Spicy Black Beans* topped with salsa and homemade guacamole

S: 2 clementines and fresh pineapple

Day 6

B: Green Smoothie,* 2 boiled eggs, and flax seed crackers with almond butter

L: Brown rice and steamed veggies

S: Green Smoothie,* 1 apple, and a handful of raw almonds

D: Simple Salmon with Ginger,* plus Lemony Quinoa with Pine Nuts and Spinach*

S: Red Velvet Smoothie*

Day 7

B: Healthy Hot and Spicy Cocoa,* plus Steel-Cut Oats with Berries and Flax Seeds*

L: Simple Salmon with Ginger,* brown rice, and steamed veggies

S: Apple with peanut butter and a handful of homemade trail mix (shredded coconut, raw almonds, unsalted peanuts, dried cranberries, sesame seeds, raisins)

D: Vibrant Veggie Soup,* Sliced Brussels Sprouts with Slivered Almonds and Dates,* roasted squash, and Kale Chips*

S: Frozen banana blended with strawberries, blueberries, and almond milk

Day 8

B: Pumpkin Smoothie,* 2 boiled eggs, and smoked salmon

L: Quinoa Tabbouleh*

S: Dried mango and a handful of raw almonds

D: Escarole with White Beans* and brown rice

S: Grapes

Day 9

B: Gluten-free granola with almond milk, strawberries, and blueberries

L: Butternut Squash Soup with Kale* and flax seed crackers

S: 1 apple and 1 pear

D: Curried chicken, brown rice, plus Curried Cauliflower and Chickpea Stew*, plus brown rice

Day 10

B: Scrambled eggs and bacon, oat scone, and freshly made green juice (kale, spinach, and green apple)

L: Mixed green salad

S: 2 navel oranges

D: Vegetable and Lentil Soup,* plus corn chips and homemade guacamole

S: Healthy Homemade Energy Bar*

A Final Note

It can be hard to prioritize long-term health and wellness because you don't usually see the results of your efforts right away. Actually, though, you're given regular status reports about your health every time you go to the bathroom. Your stool is one of the best indicators of your overall health. Not only can it provide important clues about the cause of your bloating, but it's also a reflection of whether you're putting in the right fuel to keep your digestive engine running smoothly.

It seems fitting that we're going to end this book with a quick but careful look at what happens at the end of the marvelous and complex GI superhighway.

THE ULTIMATE DETOX

A good bowel movement is the ultimate detox. Every time you eliminate stool, you're ridding your body of toxins, unwanted bacteria, and other waste products not meant to be hanging around inside you. If you have great bowel movements on a regular basis, you know exactly what I'm talking about—you feel cleansed, light, tight, and bright. If you don't feel that way, I hope this book has given you a lot to look forward to. Not evacuating in a timely manner exposes your colon to toxins in the stool for longer than necessary, which will bloat you and bog you down. It also sends mixed messages to your brain and your GI tract, which often leads to bowel confusion and inefficient emptying down the road.

TURN AROUND AND TAKE A LOOK

Since good bowel movements are an indicator of good health, you need to pay close attention to what your stool may be telling you. The best way to do that is to literally turn around and take a look at it. What you see will give you important feedback to improve your digestive health. It might even save your life, tipping you off to the early signs of colon cancer, liver disease, and infection. Are you dehydrated? Have a parasite? Pancreas problems? Bacteria out of balance? Concerned about diabetes? Not getting enough greens? Eating too much meat? Thyroid out of whack? It all comes out in the bowl. Your stool gives you crucial information to help you make changes that will nourish you from the inside out.

Five Factors for Stool Nirvana

How can you figure out what your stool is telling you, and how do you know when you've achieved what I call stool nirvana? Here are five essential factors that you should be assessing.

COLOR

- Bile and bilirubin pigment from dead red blood cells give stool its characteristic brown color.
- Pale chalky stool can be a sign of liver disease or clogged bile ducts and is often accompanied by dark urine as the bile gets excreted through the kidneys instead of the digestive tract.
- Yellow stool may mean a parasite like giardia or excess fat in the stool because of a pancreas that's not secreting enough enzymes.
- Green stool can be the result of *Clostridium difficile* infection or antibiotics.
- Red stool occurs with bleeding from the colon or eating beets.
- Black stool usually signifies bleeding from higher in the GI tract or from an iron supplement.
- A lighter brown color may mean not enough deeply pigmented leafy greens.
- Blue food coloring can actually turn your stool blue.

Stool nirvana: a deep brown color that looks like melted chocolate.

CONSISTENCY

Stool is 75 percent water, and dehydration is one of the commonest causes of a hard stool that's difficult to pass. You may not feel thirsty until you're already very dehydrated, so you need to make sure you're drinking at least a liter of pure water daily to keep your stool moist and easy to pass. Here are a few more tips:

- Plant fiber in fruits, vegetables, and beans adds bulk to your stool, making it easier for your colon to push it out.
- A kale and berry smoothie in the morning, split pea soup with a salad for lunch, and lentils and brown rice for dinner will give your stool amazing bulk and an ideal consistency.
- Stool that's too loose can be a sign of inflammation in the colon or infection with a virus, bacterium, or parasite.
- Diabetes causes loose stool when the nerves that control motility of the GI tract are affected, but it can also slow transit down and cause constipation and hard stool.
- An underactive thyroid is associated with hard stool and an overactive thyroid with loose stool.
- Medications can affect stool consistency, with narcotic pain relievers typically causing hard stool and antibiotics, magnesium-containing antacids, and diuretics causing diarrhea.
- Loose stool can also be a sign of lactose intolerance or food allergies.

Stool nirvana: a soft, bulky stool that sends a strong signal when you need to go and exits easily but is not so loose that it leaks out.

CLARITY

Bits of corn, lettuce, or other vegetable matter in the stool represent undigested cellulose and are a normal and healthy sign of a plant-based diet. People with inflammatory conditions like Crohn's or ulcerative colitis may have lots of undigested food particles in their stool because of malabsorption. In those situations there are usually additional symptoms such as weight loss, diarrhea, blood in the stool, or abdominal pain. Oily stools that float can be a sign of fat malabsorption from problems with the pancreas, liver, or gallbladder.

Stool nirvana: a little plant matter in your stool within twenty-four hours of eating it and a stool that sinks to the bottom of the bowl and doesn't float.

CUT

Pencil-thin stools can be a sign of colon cancer, diverticulosis, or inflammation in the colon. Small pebble-type stools are characteristic of diverticulosis and represent casts of diverticular potholes where the stool has been sitting. Not enough fiber in your diet can also result in pebbly stools. Stool that has been sitting in your colon a long time waiting to come out may form layers of varying colors and may be large and painful to pass. Premature squeezing of your anal sphincter may pinch off your stool before it all gets a chance to exit, giving it a sausage on a string appearance.

Stool nirvana: a thick stool the diameter of your wrist, several inches long.

CLEANUP

A stool that leaves no messy residue on exit, what I like to call the "clean wipe," is characteristic of a very high-fiber diet. The ideal stool is virtually odorless and requires no room deodorizer afterward, although cruciferous vegetables like cabbage, broccoli, and cauliflower, some types of beans, and dried fruits can cause smelly gas because of incomplete digestion and additional fermentation by bacteria. Foul-smelling stool may be a result of bacterial overgrowth; inflammation in the GI tract; infection; too many sulfur-containing foods, chemicals, or artificial flavoring in food; lactose intolerance; or too much processed meat in your diet.

Stool nirvana: an odorless stool with a clean wipe and no messy residue.

I hope I've convinced you that turning around and taking a look is worthwhile and important. If you do it regularly, you may not need to come see me!

Appendix: Gutbliss Recipes

Organic fruit and vegetables are preferred when available. If you cannot find BPA-free cans, use freshly cooked beans (see "Gutbliss Solutions for Good Gas" on page 46) and vegetables whenever possible.

BREAKFAST IDEAS*

*NOTE: For additional ideas for smoothies, see the "Custom Smoothie Guide" in the "Snacks and Treats" section (see pages 269–71).

Green Smoothie

Drinking your fresh fruit and vegetables can sometimes be more convenient than eating them, particularly when they're combined in this delicious and nutritious smoothie that works for breakfast or lunch, or as an anytime snack. The pineapple and papaya are full of digestive enzymes that help break down protein, and the nutrients and fiber in the greens will keep your good bacteria happy and healthy.

SERVES 4

1 cup almond milk or coconut milk
1 banana, sliced and frozen ahead of time

1 cup raw spinach, washed

1 cup raw kale, washed (central stem removed)

1 cup sliced fresh pineapple or papaya

❊ Place all of the ingredients in a blender and blend at high speed for 2 minutes until a smooth liquid consistency. Drink immediately after blending.

Pumpkin Smoothie

With the nostalgic flavors of a pumpkin pie, this smoothie will become your fall favorite. Pumpkin is high in antioxidants and a great source of energy to keep you fueled throughout the day. This smoothie is also an excellent precursor to winter with both the warming and anti-inflammatory properties of cinnamon, ginger, and nutmeg. For an added boost of spice and flavor, garnish with a cinnamon stick.

SERVES 4

½ cup pureed pumpkin

1 cup almond milk or coconut milk

1 banana, sliced and frozen ahead of time

1 carrot, chopped (optional)

1 scoop of plant-based vanilla protein powder (optional)

½ teaspoon vanilla extract or powdered vanilla bean

1 sliver fresh ginger root

Nutmeg and cinnamon to taste

1 cinnamon stick for garnish (optional)

Note: For additional sweetness, add 1 chopped, pitted date.

❊ Place all of the ingredients except the cinnamon stick in a blender and blend at high speed for 2 minutes until it reaches a smooth liquid consistency. Garnish with the cinnamon stick, if desired. Sip, savor, and enjoy.

Dr. Chutkan's Magic Smoothie

My magic smoothie is full of live food and bloat-busting fiber and is a great way to start the day. It's an outstanding alternative to breakfast cereal that's been sitting in a box for months or pancakes or muffins whose main ingre-

dient is sugar. I recommend having this smoothie every day while you're on the plan, in the morning for breakfast or as a snack later in the day.

MAKES 2 LARGE SERVINGS

1 sliced ripe banana

2 cups organic mixed berries

1 cup raw spinach, kale, collards, or chard, washed (central stem removed for kale/collards/chard)

1 tablespoon ground psyllium husk

1 tablespoon ground flax seed

1 cup crushed ice

1 cup almond milk, coconut milk, or coconut water

✻ In a blender bowl, combine all of the ingredients. Blend well and drink immediately.

Morning Quinoa

Quinoa was first domesticated by the Incas thousands of years ago, and although it's thought of as a grain, it's actually a leafy green vegetable like spinach that's cultivated for its seeds. It's a great source of plant protein (one cup has about 8 grams) and is easily digestible and gluten-free. It has a slightly nutty taste, similar to brown rice. This protein-packed nutritional powerhouse is also high in magnesium, phosphorus, and iron. Start your day on the right note and enjoy the benefits of a steady flow of energy.

SERVES 4 TO 6

1 cup quinoa

2 cups water

¼ cup diced yellow squash

¼ cup thinly sliced carrot rounds

¼ cup raisins

¼ cup chopped walnuts

¼ cup whole or ground sesame seeds

¼ cup coconut milk, almond milk, or hemp milk

Sprinkle of cinnamon

HOW TO COOK THE QUINOA: In a fine-mesh strainer, rinse the quinoa well with cool water until the water runs clear. This will remove the outer coating, which can give it a bitter taste. In a saucepan, bring the water to a boil over medium-high heat. Add the quinoa, reduce the heat, and bring the mixture to a light boil for 5 minutes, and then simmer, covered, for an additional 15 minutes. Remove from the heat and let stand for 5 minutes, covered. After 5 minutes, remove the lid and fluff the quinoa gently with a fork. Serve.

❊ For this recipe, when the quinoa first starts to simmer, stir in the squash, carrots, raisins, walnuts, and sesame seeds. Add the plant-based milk after cooking, to achieve the desired consistency. Sprinkle with cinnamon.

Steel-Cut Oats with Berries and Flax Seeds

Oats contain antioxidants and lignans, which protect against cancer and help stabilize blood sugar levels. Steel-cut oats are minimally processed and also don't have the added sugar of most brands of instant oatmeal. If you don't have time to cook this in the morning, simply make a batch in advance to enjoy it in single-size portions throughout the week.

SERVES 4

1 cup steel-cut oats
3 cups water
1 tablespoon ground flax seeds
2 cups organic blueberries, raspberries, and/or strawberries
Drizzle of flax seed oil (optional)
Nutrient-dense toppings (see "Delicious Variations for Toppings" below) (optional)

❊ In a saucepan, combine the oats, water, and flax seeds, stir briefly, and bring to a boil over medium-high heat. Reduce the heat to low, cover, and simmer for 20 to 25 minutes, or until the oats are tender and the liquid is almost totally absorbed. Top with the berries, drizzle with flax seed oil, if desired, and serve. Or top with your other favorite nutrient-dense toppings, such as bananas and walnuts, or coconut, cinnamon, and pitted dates.

❊ For a quicker version, soak the oats in the water in a 2-quart saucepan for 8 to 12 hours or overnight. In the morning, add the ground flax seeds and bring to a boil, reduce the heat to low, and simmer, stirring constantly, for 5 minutes. Top with the berries, drizzle with flax seed oil, if desired, and serve. Or top with your other favorite nutrient-dense toppings.

Delicious Variations for Toppings:
Blueberries and walnuts
Sliced banana and walnuts
Apricots and almonds
Apple, pecans, and cinnamon
Dried cranberries and almonds
Pear, ginger, and flax seeds
Shredded coconut and sliced banana
Coconut, cinnamon, and pitted dates

SOUPS

Split Pea Soup/Dal

Split peas are a member of the legume family and are a great source of fiber that can help to lower your cholesterol and improve bowel regularity. This versatile dish can be made as a liquid for soup or, with a thicker consistency, for dal that can be served over rice or quinoa.

SERVES 6 TO 8
1 pound yellow split peas, rinsed and drained
6 cups low-sodium organic chicken or vegetable broth for dal, 8 cups for
     soup
3 large cloves garlic, minced
1-2 cups coconut milk (1 cup for dal, 2 cups for soup) (optional)
3 scallions, chopped
1 jalapeño pepper, diced
1 sprig of fresh thyme
½ teaspoon cumin
1 teaspoon curry powder
Freshly ground black pepper to taste

❖ Boil the split peas in the chicken or vegetable broth with the garlic until the peas are soft (about 1 hour). Add additional broth or water as needed to keep the mixture liquid. Add the coconut milk, if using, and boil for an additional 10 minutes. Add the scallions, jalapeños, and thyme and cook for 10 minutes more. Remove from the heat and blend with a handheld stick blender or puree in a food processor. Return to the heat and cook an additional 30 minutes. Season with curry powder, cumin, and freshly ground black pepper to taste. Serve.

Butternut Squash Soup with Kale

The savory roasted vegetables and herbs in this recipe combine beautifully to create a smooth, creamy, and nourishing soup. The addition of kale tops off this bowl filled with nutrients from vitamin A to zinc. Serve garnished with toasted pumpkin seeds.

SERVES 8

4 cups butternut squash, peeled and coarsely chopped
2 cups sweet potatoes, peeled and coarsely chopped
3 tablespoons olive oil
3 large cloves garlic, minced
1 tablespoon fresh rosemary
1 tablespoon fresh sage
1 tablespoon fresh thyme
1 medium onion, coarsely chopped
2 large carrots, coarsely chopped
2 red bell peppers, coarsely chopped
6 cups low-sodium organic vegetable broth
3 cups raw kale, washed, central stem removed, and sliced into strips
Freshly ground black pepper to taste
Sprigs of fresh herbs (rosemary, thyme, oregano) or pumpkin seeds for
    garnish

❖ Preheat oven to 375°F. Place the squash and sweet potatoes in a large roasting pan and toss with the olive oil, garlic, rosemary, sage, and thyme. Roast uncovered in the oven for 30 minutes. Add the onions, carrots, and bell peppers. Roast for an additional 20 to 30 minutes, or until the vegetables are golden brown. Remove the pan from the oven and place the roasted vegetables in a large stockpot. Add the vegetable broth. Heat over medium-high heat until the squash begins to soften. Turn the heat off and blend the soup with a handheld stick blender (see Note below). Add the sliced kale to the blended soup and cook over medium heat uncovered for 2 to 3 minutes, or until the kale wilts. Season with freshly ground black pepper. Serve in bowls and garnish with a sprig of fresh herbs or pumpkin seeds.

Note: If a stick blender is not available, use a food processor or high-speed blender after allowing the soup to cool slightly, but while still hot.

Vibrant Veggie Soup

This sumptuous soup is great to have on hand and enjoy any time of day. It makes a nourishing snack as well as a filling addition to any meal. If you have a limited amount of time to prepare your food during the week, this is an easy way to guarantee that you get your veggies every day.

SERVES 8

2 tablespoons olive oil

1 yellow or sweet onion, diced

1 clove garlic, diced

5 celery stalks, sliced into ½-inch segments

4 carrots, sliced into thin rounds

2 tablespoons fresh herbs, chopped (parsley, oregano, and/or thyme)

4 cups homemade or store-bought low-sodium organic vegetable stock

1 to 2 cups water, depending on desired thickness

One 28-ounce can/carton diced tomatoes

One 6-ounce can tomato paste

6 cups vegetables, chopped (such as broccoli, asparagus, red bell peppers, yellow squash, zucchini, green beans)

3 cups fresh raw spinach leaves, washed

Freshly ground black pepper to taste

Red pepper flakes (optional, but recommended for an additional kick)

❖ Heat the olive oil in a soup pot and add the onions, garlic, celery, and carrots. Sauté the vegetables for about 5 to 10 minutes, until lightly browned. Then add the fresh herbs and stir to coat the vegetables. Add the vegetable stock, water, diced tomatoes, and tomato paste. Mix thoroughly and stir in the chopped vegetables. Bring to a boil, reduce the heat to low, and simmer, covered, for 30 to 35 minutes, or until the vegetables are soft. Turn off the heat and add the spinach leaves. Cover the pot for 5 minutes to allow the spinach to steam. Remove the cover. Season the soup with freshly ground black pepper and red pepper flakes, if desired. Ladle into bowls and serve.

Moroccan Gazpacho Soup

This chilled Middle Eastern tomato-based soup is refreshing, spicy, and flavorful, and it can also be made in advance and served on a warm summer day. You get the perfect combination of spices that offer anti-inflammatory benefits along with a huge dose of lycopene from the fresh tomatoes.

SERVES 4

4 cloves garlic, minced

2½ teaspoons paprika

1½ teaspoons ground cumin

Pinch of cayenne pepper

4 teaspoons olive oil, plus oil for drizzling

2½ pounds tomatoes, diced and cut into 1-inch cubes

1 tablespoon white wine vinegar

Juice of 1 lemon

2 tablespoons water

¼ cup chopped celery or cilantro for garnish

❖ In a small sauté pan, combine the garlic, paprika, cumin, cayenne, and olive oil. Cook over low heat, stirring constantly, for 2 minutes. Remove from the heat and let cool. Next, blend the tomatoes in a food processor. Stir in the spice mixture, vinegar, lemon juice, and water with the tomatoes. Refrigerate until cold. Serve garnished with chopped celery or cilantro and a drizzle of olive oil.

Vegetable and Lentil Soup

Lentil soup can be very satisfying in the colder winter months. For a heartier meal, serve over basmati rice, or, to boost the nutritional value of the meal, add in some kale or spinach at the end. The soup keeps in the refrigerator for days, and it is a meal in itself.

SERVES 12

2 tablespoons olive oil

3 large celery stalks, chopped into ½-inch segments

2 large carrots, chopped into thin rounds

1 large onion, chopped

3 cloves garlic, chopped

1½ teaspoons chopped fresh rosemary leaves

1½ teaspoons dried oregano

8 cups low-sodium organic vegetable or chicken broth

One 28-ounce can diced tomatoes, including juice

2 cups (about 11 ounces) green lentils, rinsed

⅓ cup chopped fresh Italian parsley leaves (about half a bunch)

Freshly ground black pepper

❖ Heat the olive oil in a large, heavy pot over medium-high heat. Add the celery, carrots, onions, garlic, rosemary, and oregano. Sauté until the onions are translucent, about 8 minutes. Add the vegetable or chicken broth and tomatoes with their juice. Bring the soup to a boil. Reduce the heat to medium-low, cover, and simmer until the vegetables are just tender, stirring occasionally, about 30 minutes. Add the lentils. Cover and continue simmering until the lentils are softened, about 1 hour. Stir in the parsley. Season the soup to taste with freshly ground black pepper. Ladle into bowls and serve.

Blended Green Soup

Have you ever made a soup in less than ten minutes? This blended soup is an excellent way to fuel your body without having to slave over the stove. Blending your greens ensures that the tough cell membranes are broken down so that you start nourishing your body with the very first sip.

SERVES 4

3 cups chopped raw spinach, washed

3 stalks celery, chopped

1 sprig of oregano

1 red bell pepper, chopped

1 large avocado, sliced

1 cucumber, chopped

1 jalapeño pepper, diced

Juice of 1 lime

2 cups water

✻ Combine all of the ingredients in the bowl of a blender. Blend and enjoy!

Curried Cauliflower and Chickpea Stew

Cauliflower by itself is often considered bland, but the addition of curry, garlic, and ginger makes this dish a tasty part of any anti-inflammatory diet. This soup is perfect on its own or can be served with brown rice and steamed greens for a complete and satisfying meal.

SERVES 4

1 head cauliflower

1 medium yellow onion, thinly sliced

2 cloves garlic, minced

1-inch piece of fresh ginger, peeled and cut into thin slices

1 tablespoon grapeseed oil

2 carrots, sliced into thin rounds

1 tablespoon curry powder

2 cups low-sodium organic vegetable stock

1½ cups chopped tomatoes with their juices

1½ cups cooked chickpeas

2 tablespoons raisins

Freshly ground black pepper

Chopped fresh basil

✻ Wash the cauliflower and remove the outer leaves and inner stems. Cut the florets into bite-size pieces and set aside. In a Dutch oven over medium-high heat, sauté the onions, garlic, and ginger in the grapeseed oil until lightly browned. Add the carrots and cook for an additional 2 minutes. Add the curry powder, vegetable stock, tomatoes, and chickpeas. Bring the soup to a boil, then reduce the heat to medium-low and bring the soup to a simmer before folding in the cauliflower and raisins. Cover and cook until the cauliflower is soft, about 7 minutes. Season with freshly ground black pepper to taste. Garnish with chopped basil and serve.

SALADS

Rainbow Salad

A balanced diet contains the full spectrum of colors. The way to create a delicious and nourishing salad packed with plant-derived phytonutrients is to represent each color of the rainbow. Go for variety and try to add tastes and colors that have been missing from your diet. Some examples of ingredients to choose from:

Red fruits and vegetables: red bell peppers, tomatoes, rhubarb, berries, pomegranate seeds, red onions, pink grapefruit, beets, radishes

Orange/yellow fruits and vegetables: carrots, orange bell peppers, pumpkin, papayas, apricots, squash, pineapples, sweet corn, sweet potatoes, mangoes

Green fruits and vegetables: celery, romaine lettuce, arugula, kale, dandelion greens, spinach, mixed greens, sprouts, broccoli, roasted Brussels sprouts, zucchini, green onions, peas, avocados

Black/purple fruits and vegetables: roasted eggplant, purple cabbage, figs, plums, blueberries, blackberries

White fruits and vegetables: cauliflower, jicama, ginger root, mushrooms, garlic, onions, scallions

Heart-healthy oils: Flax seed oil, walnut oil, olive oil, avocado oil (these oils add in "good" fats)

Fresh herbs: Parsley, cilantro, basil, oregano

Protein: Plant-based protein (legumes, nuts, seeds) or animal-based protein (chicken breast, turkey breast, fish, shellfish, lean meat)

❖ Assemble all ingredients in a large bowl (a glass bowl is fun, so you can enjoy all the colors). Be creative! Season the salad with fresh herbs and homemade vinaigrette. This salad can be stored undressed in a well-sealed container in the fridge for several days. You can use handfuls at a time in different ways, including: add chopped chicken or turkey; toss in cooked lentils; drizzle with olive oil and balsamic vinegar; stuff into a corn tortilla; or wilt into a breakfast omelet.

MAINS AND SIDES

Quinoa Tabbouleh

This is a modern take on an old favorite. Traditionally, tabbouleh is made with bulgur wheat, but this version has quinoa, which is not only gluten-free but also contains a healthy dose of plant-based protein. Tabbouleh is satisfying as a main dish served on a bed of greens and can be made in advance for an easy on-the-go meal.

SERVES 8

1 cup quinoa

2 cups water or low-sodium organic vegetable broth

1 cup cucumbers, peeled and chopped

1 cup fresh parsley, chopped

¼ cup fresh mint, chopped

1 cup grape tomatoes, quartered

½ cup scallions, chopped

Freshly ground black pepper to taste

¼ cup olive oil

¼ cup fresh lemon juice

1 teaspoon minced garlic

✳ In a saucepan, cook the quinoa in the water or vegetable broth according to the directions in the Morning Quinoa recipe (see pages 249–50). Chill the quinoa thoroughly in the fridge for at least 1 hour. In a bowl, combine the chilled quinoa, cucumbers, parsley, mint, grape tomatoes, and scallions. Season with freshly ground black pepper to taste. In a separate bowl, whisk the olive oil, lemon juice, and garlic until blended. Add to the quinoa and veggies and mix until thoroughly combined. Chill before serving.

Lemony Quinoa with Pine Nuts and Spinach

Quinoa has the highest nutritional profile and cooks the fastest of all the grains (while it's technically a seed, we consume it like a grain). Quinoa is the only plant-based food that has all eight essential amino acids, making it a complete protein. In addition to being gluten-free, quinoa is high in B vitamins, iron, zinc, potassium, calcium, and vitamin E. Spinach and parsley enhance the nutritional benefits of this dish.

SERVES 8

1 cup quinoa

2 cups water

2 cups raw spinach, washed

½ cup pine nuts

¼ cup olive oil, plus a dab for the pine nuts

½ cup golden raisins

2 teaspoons freshly grated lemon zest

½ cup chopped fresh flat-leaf parsley

¼ cup fresh lemon juice

1 teaspoon ground cumin

Freshly ground black pepper to taste

�֎ Preheat the oven to 325°F. In a saucepan, cook the quinoa with the water according to the directions in the Morning Quinoa recipe. While the quinoa is cooking, slice the spinach into thin strips. Brush the pine nuts with a dab of olive oil, place them on a baking sheet, and bake them in the oven until lightly toasted, about 10 minutes. Transfer the warm, cooked quinoa to a serving bowl and add the toasted pine nuts, raisins, lemon zest, and parsley. Place the sliced raw spinach on top of the quinoa. In a separate bowl, whisk together the lemon juice and cumin. Slowly add in the remaining ¼ cup olive oil to form a paste. Pour the dressing over the quinoa mixture, making certain to moisten all of the ingredients. Add freshly ground black pepper to taste. Serve this nourishing and delicious dish warm or at room temperature.

Braised Baby Bok Choy

Sometimes you may need a break from kale. Bok choy, also referred to as an Asian green, is a mild-tasting member of the cabbage family. Use this recipe as a guide to cooking delicious greens. For a change, swap out the bok choy for any of your favorite leafies.

SERVES 2 TO 4

1 cup low-sodium organic vegetable broth
3 tablespoons olive oil
¾ pound baby bok choy, trimmed
½ teaspoon sesame oil
Freshly ground black pepper to taste

❊ In a large, deep, heavy skillet, combine the vegetable broth and olive oil over medium heat and bring them to a simmer. Arrange the bok choy evenly in the skillet and simmer covered, until tender, about 5 minutes. Transfer the bok choy with tongs to a serving dish and cover to keep warm. Increase the heat to high and boil the broth mixture until reduced to about ¼ cup, then stir in the sesame oil and freshly ground black pepper to taste. Pour the mixture over the greens.

Noah's Asian Turkey Sliders

Elise's son, Noah, came up with this tasty recipe after trying to figure out how to re-create the flavor of pot stickers but in a healthier way. Serve with brown rice or over a bed of greens.

SERVES 4 TO 6

1 pound ground turkey breast
3 teaspoons finely grated ginger root
2 cloves garlic, chopped
2 egg whites
1 large carrot, finely grated
2 tablespoons gluten-free soy sauce
2 teaspoons sesame oil
1 tablespoon freshly minced cilantro (optional)

3 green onions, minced

Freshly ground black pepper to taste

Vegetable oil for the griddle or pan

❀ Combine the turkey, ginger, garlic, egg whites, carrots, soy sauce, sesame oil, cilantro if using, green onions, and freshly ground black pepper to taste in a medium bowl. Form the mixture into patties about 1½ to 2 inches in diameter. Place the patties on a lightly oiled griddle or in a lightly oiled pan and cook over medium-high heat for about 7 minutes per side, or until cooked through. Serve immediately.

Lemony Roasted Chicken

Every chef has a version of a whole roasted chicken. The secret ingredient to this tasty chicken is the lemon juice. It seals in the bird's natural juices and helps crisp and brown the skin. Use an organic free-range chicken if possible.

SERVES 4

1 chicken, 2 to 4 pounds

1 lemon

1 medium onion, peeled

2 cloves garlic

2 to 3 sprigs each of fresh rosemary, sage, and thyme

Poultry seasoning

Freshly ground black pepper to taste

½ cup low-sodium organic chicken broth

❀ Preheat the oven to 450°F. Rinse the chicken, pat it dry, and remove and discard the giblets. Cut the lemon in half and squeeze the juice onto the skin. Place the onion, garlic cloves, and one each of the fresh sprigs of herbs in the cavity. Season the cavity with freshly ground black pepper to taste. Generously season the outside of the chicken with freshly ground pepper and poultry seasoning.

❀ Place the chicken on a rack in a heavy roasting pan. Pour the chicken broth into the pan and roast uncovered for 30 minutes. Reduce the heat to 375°F and continue to roast for at least 1 hour more, or until the juices run clear. Remove the chicken from the oven and let stand for 5 minutes before carving. Garnish with the remaining sprigs of fresh herbs.

Escarole with White Beans

Escarole often has a bitter taste, but with the flavor of the white beans and spice from the garlic, this escarole can't be beat. Escarole is filled with fiber, folic acid, vitamin A, and vitamin K. The white beans add a nutritional boost of plant-based protein.

SERVES 4

2 tablespoons olive oil
2 cloves garlic, sliced
1 head escarole, washed and chopped
One 15-ounce can great northern white beans, rinsed and drained, or 1½ cups cooked great northern white beans
Freshly ground black pepper to taste

✻ In a large sauté pan, heat the olive oil hot enough so that when you add the garlic, it sizzles as it hits the pan. Slowly add the escarole. Sauté for 3 to 5 minutes, or until wilted. Add the beans, turn off the heat, and mix well. Season with freshly ground black pepper to taste. Dig into this hearty and tasty dish of greens!

Simple Salmon with Ginger

Salmon is often revered for its omega-3 fatty acids. The combination of salmon, ginger, and plum vinegar in this recipe creates a fresh, light flavor with a subtle zing.

SERVES 2

1 tablespoon coconut oil
¼ cup water
2 teaspoons freshly grated ginger

1 tablespoon plum vinegar

2 wild salmon fillets (4 ounces each)

Lemon or lime slices for garnish

❄ Make a marinade by combining the coconut oil, water, ginger, and plum vinegar. Place the fish in a shallow baking dish, cover with the marinade, and refrigerate for at least 30 minutes, up to 12 hours in the refrigerator. Set aside a few tablespoons of the marinade to use for basting and discard the rest. Preheat the broiler. Broil the fish, skin side down, for 8 to 10 minutes, until the flesh is opaque and flakes easily when a fork is inserted. Baste with the remaining marinade once or twice while broiling. Serve garnished with lemon or lime slices.

Roasted Fish in Tomato Sauce

This recipe transforms a mild white fish into a flavorful creation. It is easy to prepare and looks beautiful right out of the oven.

SERVES 4

2 tablespoons olive oil, plus enough to coat the baking dish

4 white fish fillets, such as cod, flounder, snapper, or sea bass (6 ounces each)

1 yellow onion, finely chopped

2 cloves garlic, finely minced

6 plum tomatoes, seeded and chopped

Freshly ground black pepper to taste

3 tablespoons finely chopped Italian parsley

2 tablespoons fresh basil, sliced into thin strips

1 tablespoon finely chopped fresh thyme

❄ Preheat the oven to 450°F. Oil a large baking dish. Arrange the fish in a single layer in the prepared baking dish. Heat the 2 tablespoons olive oil in a saucepan. Add the onions and sauté for 8 to 10 minutes, until the onions are tender and translucent. Add the garlic and sauté for 1 minute more. Stir in the chopped tomatoes and cook over low heat until the sauce thickens, about 15 minutes. Season the sauce to taste with freshly ground black pepper. Stir in half of the parsley, basil, and thyme, and simmer the sauce for 2 minutes more. Spoon the sauce on top of the fish and bake the fish in the preheated oven for 10 to 12 minutes, depending on the thickness of the fish. The flesh should be opaque and flake easily with a fork when done. Remove from oven and sprinkle with the remaining parsley, basil, and thyme before serving.

Baked Cod with Spicy Peppers

This simple fish dish is not only delicious and easy to prepare, it's also loaded with a variety of spices that have anti-inflammatory benefits.

SERVES 4

1 medium poblano pepper
½ jalapeño pepper
2 tablespoons olive oil
2 cloves garlic
1 shallot
¼ teaspoon cayenne pepper
Pinch of sea salt
1½ pounds cod fillets

✤ Preheat the oven to 350°F. Wash and dry the poblano and jalapeño peppers and rub them with a small amount of olive oil. Roast the peppers on a baking sheet in the oven until they're soft and the skin is blistering. Remove the peppers from the oven, cover, and let sit for 5 minutes. Peel away the skin and remove the seeds and stems. Combine the roasted peppers, remaining olive oil, garlic, shallot, cayenne, and sea salt in food processor and puree until smooth.

✤ Cover a cookie sheet with parchment paper, place the cod fillets on the sheet, and spread the puree of roasted peppers evenly over the cod fillet tops and sides. Bake for 20 to 30 minutes, or until fish flakes easily when tested with a fork.

Sliced Brussels Sprouts with Slivered Almonds and Dates

You probably turned your nose up at these as a kid. Now it's time to make amends and enjoy this close relative of the cabbage. Brussels sprouts are loaded with a hefty dose of vitamin K, which helps with calcium absorption. Slice and sauté the Brussels sprouts, and then mix with shallots, dates, and slivered almonds for a winning combination.

SERVES 4 TO 6

2 tablespoons olive oil

2 large shallots, minced

1 pound Brussels sprouts, cored and sliced

Freshly ground black pepper to taste

Juice and zest of ½ lemon

¼ cup slivered almonds, toasted

¼ cup Medjool dates, pitted and chopped

❖ In a large saucepan, heat 1 tablespoon of the olive oil and sauté the shallots for 2 to 3 minutes, until golden brown. Remove the shallots, add the remaining tablespoon olive oil, and cook the Brussels sprouts for 4 to 5 minutes, until slightly browned. Season with freshly ground black pepper to taste. Mix the cooked shallots into the sprouts. Add the lemon juice and lemon zest. Toss in the almonds and dates.

Spicy Black Beans

These spicy beans can be eaten as a main dish over rice or on their own, and they also make a tasty side dish. They keep well in the freezer and can be blended with low-sodium organic chicken or vegetable broth to create a hearty black bean soup.

SERVES 6 TO 8

1 pound dried black beans

1 tablespoon olive oil

½ cup finely chopped onion

½ cup finely chopped carrots

3 cloves garlic, chopped

2 bay leaves

1 teaspoon ground cumin

1 tablespoon Worcestershire sauce

1 tablespoon balsamic vinegar

1 teaspoon Italian seasoning

Dash of cayenne pepper

Squeeze of lemon or lime juice

❊ Place the dried beans in a bowl and cover with water (about 3 inches past the level of the beans). Let the beans soak for at least 1 hour or overnight. In a large saucepan, heat the olive oil and sauté the onions, carrots, and garlic until tender, about 10 minutes. Drain the water from the beans and add the beans to the onions, carrots, and garlic, plus enough water to generously cover everything in the saucepan by at least 1 inch. Add the bay leaves. Cover and let the beans simmer on low heat for 45 minutes, but keep stirring frequently and add water as necessary to make sure the beans don't burn. Add the cumin, Worcestershire sauce, vinegar, Italian seasoning, and cayenne. Let the mixture cook for at least 2 hours uncovered, stirring regularly and adding water as needed. Add the lemon or lime juice. Cook until the sauce has thickened and the beans are soft (about an additional 30 minutes). Discard the bay leaves before serving.

SNACKS AND TREATS

Kale Chips

This recipe is easy to make and can add a healthy dose of crunch along with chlorophyll, vitamins, minerals, and phytonutrients. Specifically, kale is rich in potent cancer-fighting substances, is loaded with bone-building vitamin K, and has one of the highest antioxidant levels of all vegetables. Did I mention that these chips taste good too?

SERVES 4 TO 6

6 cups raw kale (about 2 bunches), rinsed with (central stem removed)

1 tablespoon apple cider vinegar

2 tablespoons olive oil

Sea salt to taste (but just a little!)

❊ Preheat oven to 350°F. Cut the kale leaves into 2- to 3-inch pieces. Mix the vinegar, olive oil, and salt in a large bowl. Add the kale and mix by hand to evenly coat all of the leaves. Place the kale leaves on parchment-lined baking sheets (I like to use parchment paper for easy cleanup) and bake until the kale leaves are crispy, about 5 to 10 minutes.

Note: Baking time may vary depending on the size of your chips and desired crispness.

Spicy Roasted Chickpeas

These roasted chickpeas are the perfect addition to a salad or grain dish. The flavorful beans also work well as a snack to satisfy any craving for crunch. This dish can be made in advance and stored in an airtight container. Play around with the seasonings, but if you like very spicy, then use an entire teaspoon of cayenne pepper (instead of the paprika) and a dash of red pepper flakes.

SERVES 4

2 tablespoons olive oil

1 teaspoon Spanish smoked paprika

1 teaspoon cumin

Pinch of cayenne pepper

One 15-ounce can chickpeas, rinsed, drained, and patted dry

❋ Preheat oven to 400°F. Combine the olive oil, paprika, cumin, and cayenne in a large bowl. Add the chickpeas and toss to coat evenly. Transfer the chickpeas to a parchment-lined baking sheet and spread in a single layer. Bake for 25 to 35 minutes, until golden and crisp (stir once after 15 minutes). Remove the baking sheet from the oven. Cool, and then transfer the chickpeas to a serving dish or an airtight container for storage. This healthy snack will stay good for a few weeks in the fridge.

Red Velvet Smoothie

This flavorful treat tastes like a frozen red velvet cupcake but without the refined flour, eggs, sugar, and red dye. Enjoy this when you're craving something sweet. And for all of you chocoholics who want to channel your addiction in a healthy way, this is for you!

4 large ripe bananas, frozen and sliced

1½ cups frozen organic raspberries

2 tablespoons unsweetened (non-alkalized) cocoa powder

4 to 5 dates, pitted and chopped

½ to 1 cup almond milk, hemp milk, or other milk substitute

❊ Blend all of the ingredients in a high-powered blender until thick and creamy.

Healthy Hot and Spicy Cocoa

If you're a fan of dark, antioxidant-rich chocolate, then you'll love this sumptuously spiced, healthy hot cocoa recipe. As a bonus, the variety of warm and inviting spices offers an array of health benefits that you don't get in the more traditional versions. So forget the guilt and take a moment to relax and enjoy this deliciously decadent drink.

SERVES 1

1 cup almond milk, hemp milk, or rice milk

1½ tablespoons unsweetened (non-alkalized) cocoa powder

Splash of vanilla extract

Sprinkle of cinnamon

Sprinkle of chili powder

Sprinkle of ground nutmeg

Sprinkle of ground cloves

❊ In a saucepan over medium-low heat, heat the plant-based milk until luke-warm. Stir the cocoa powder into the warmed liquid until dissolved. Add the vanilla extract, cinnamon, chili powder, nutmeg, and cloves. Heat for another 2 minutes, stirring occasionally. Inhale the great aroma, sip, and enjoy.

Healthy Homemade Energy Bars

Energy bars are an excellent option for an on-the-go snack or to bring with you when you travel. These homemade treats also offer a quick boost after a workout. Most commercially available energy bars are loaded with sugar, a super-long list of ingredients, and added preservatives. This homemade version is packed with heart-healthy nuts, dates for natural sweetness, and antioxidant-rich cocoa powder. They are so simple to make, you don't even have to turn on the oven!

SERVES 6 TO 8

1 cup walnuts, almonds, or cashews

1 teaspoon pure vanilla extract

1⅓ cups Medjool dates, pitted

3 to 4 tablespoons cocoa powder

1 teaspoon cinnamon

Shredded coconut to sprinkle and press on top (optional)

❈ Blend the nuts, vanilla extract, dates, cocoa powder, and cinnamon in a food processor. Spread the mixture on a baking pan or cutting board. Sprinkle with shredded coconut, if desired. Cut the mixture into square or rectangular shapes. Store in the refrigerator in an airtight container for up to 10 days or freeze for up to a month.

CUSTOM SMOOTHIE GUIDE

Your smoothie repertoire is limited only by your imagination. There are lots of ways to mix and match flavors. The one thing that never changes is the big nutritional punch you get!

BASE INGREDIENTS

- Brewed herbal tea
- Coconut milk
- Coconut water
- Nut milks (almond, hazelnut, cashew)
- Rice milk
- Seed milks (hemp, sunflower, sesame)
- Vegetable juice (fresh)
- Water

SWEETENERS

- Dates
- Fruit (fresh or frozen)

FATS AND PROTEINS

- Avocado
- Chia seeds
- Coconut oil
- Flax seed oil
- Nuts (nut butters)
- Plant-based protein powder
- Seeds (ground seeds/seed butter)
- Shredded coconut

FRUITS AND GREENS

- Apple
- Avocado
- Banana (sliced/frozen)
- Berries (fresh/frozen)
- Celery
- Collards
- Cucumber
- Dandelion greens
- Kale
- Mango
- Mint
- Papaya
- Parsley
- Peach
- Pear
- Pineapple
- Plum
- Romaine lettuce
- Spinach
- Sprouts

- Swiss chard
- Watercress

- Cocoa powder (unsweetened non-alkalized)
- Ginger (fresh grated)
- Goji berries
- Spices (nutmeg, cinnamon, vanilla)

Index